THE GOOD,
the bad, &
THE HOMELY

THE GOOD,
the bad, &
THE HOMELY

*...being a casual series of essays, as grammatically correct
as I could conveniently contrive, on the practice of medicine
in general, and plastic surgery in particular, toward the end of
the second Millennium in the United States of America.*

CHARLES E. MOORE, MD

Ardor Scribendi

NEW YORK CITY

For information, write:

ARDOR SCRIBENDI

145 East 32nd Street, 10th Floor, New York, New York 10016

Telephone: 212-889-6225 Facsimile: 212-889-8268

ISBN 1-893357-03-1

Printed in the United States of America

TO MY FATHER

who showed me how I might learn to write a little

AND MY MOTHER

who showed me more than a little how I might learn to live

Nor to forget my gratitiude to A. Bernard Ackerman, MD,
and Ardor Scribendi, who made this volume possible

CONTENTS

Preface xi

Introduction xv

Apologia xxi

Preambulation xxv

THE GOOD

Introductory: The Good 3

"Practicing" Medicine: I 9

"Practicing" Medicine: II. Keeping Your Fingers in the Proper Order 14

Whales, Maybe Codfish 18

Li'l Miracle Socker 23

Phlebotomized and Other Pleasures 28

A Chart Unchained 32

Bouquets of Clichés 36

ACLS Yes 40

Clinical Diagnosis, Brilliant and Not So 44

Romancing the Stone 49

Yes, I Am a Doctor 54

Strange, the Strange Attractor 58

Organs, What Ho! 62

Solo 67

The Nose Knows 71

The Three Greatest 76

Working (a Little) for Food 82

Teaching and Learning Food 86

Refutin' Newton 92

Everything, and More, I Know about X-Rays 96

With a Fifth of Lagavulin 101

Galen Lives! 105

Universal Untruth Be Damned 109

Speaks Still the Past 114

Braveheart Amongst Us 119

Facts Are Facts, but Art Is a Mess 125

In the Real World, Image Is Money 130

The Scan Is Quicker but Art Is Thicker 133

THE BAD

Introductory: The Bad 141

Even in Vermont 144

A Humble, Homely Apology 149

Economic Credentialing and the High Cost of Kleenex 153

Letter from the Masked Man 156

Overview: the Breast 160

   Brandy, Please, a Double 166

   To Washington! Like Mr. Smith I Wish 170

   Nolo Nocere 173

   The Defense Rests, with Footnotes 177

Afterview: the Breast 182

Vegetables and Other Media Alternatives 184

Above the Law 188

Ancien Régime Syndrome 193

THE HOMELY

Introductory: The Homely 199

Requiem for a "Cookie" 201

A Touch of Tolerance 206

The Power Nap 209

"Practicing" Medicine: III. Relief of Boredom 213

Lecture Circuit 216

Doctor-Patient-Doctor Relationship 220

Stendhal Syndrome and Other Italian Symptoms: I 225

Stendhal Syndrome and Other Italian Symptoms: II 229

Polonius Resurrected 234

3:00 A.M. 238

Even Mozart Couldn't Purr 242

Elevation of Eyebrow 246

Hmm 250

Pannicular-Laparoscopic Syndromes 254

The Breath of Death 259

What's That That "Happens"? 264

The Physician as Dog 268

While We're at It 272

Finally, a Sort of Solution 276

At Least They Don't Drink 280

Choosing My Colors 284

Decorum in Rebus Adversis 288

The Complexity of Ignorance 292

An Editorial Comment 296

Thanks, Sir Francis, but No Thanks 299

Bless the Trivia, That It May Be Discarded 303

Still Looking Good! 306

The Best Toast 311

Modem Upgrade 315

Staying Loose 319

Keeping the Balance 322

On Motherhood, Indeed! 326

The Homely View 330

But Is It a Shoe? 335

End of the Beginning 339

The World Is Not Coming to an End—Not Quite Yet! 343

Death of a Countess 348

Dénouement 353

Epilogue 359

PREFACE

These essays, most of them originally published in the Journal of the Florida Medical Association, have been read to my absolute knowledge by slightly under twelve people. In any event, I have received as a result of them perhaps six of what I shall call complimentary "fan letters," all from physicians, and usually written hastily on the front or back of a blank prescription, or otherwise bit of scratch paper advertising the latest antidepressant. Given that the physician's time even yet remains at a premium, I am glad herewith to acknowledge my sincere gratitude for the kind words these ladies and gentlemen took the time to write me. I even thank a seventh writer for what must be called a missile more than a missive for his observation that I was a pompous ass, or words closely to that effect. It pleases me to report that I rather chuckled, knowing that I am at least not pompous and was yet capable of a chuckle in the face of such adversity.

Beyond these encomiums I have been accosted by three fellow physicians who have verbally, over a bowl of soup in the doctor's lounge of the hospital where I am allowed to practice, congratulated me on this or that essay. I have always met their kind remarks with a certain modest diffidence, which did not truly do justice to my gratitude for them. We physicians and surgeons yet strive, and all the more so given the climate of these hard-pressed times, to appear to rise above mere circumstance. It is doubtless a defense of sorts, but tends even now to be misinterpreted as pomposity.

Allow me to beg, if you yourself are reading any of these essays while sipping your soup, the same tolerance towards them that you might proffer, indeed, that soup. There is no such thing as a "perfect soup," and the glory of any soup lies in its almost arbitrary and sometimes accidental interminglings of essential flavors, making it unique, and therefore of a particular value. So, too, an essay. In this world of ever greater conformities, both essays and soups should be permitted a considerable latitude in their ingredients and presentation, to be savored, or not, with an open mind. Having done so, one can then exercise the powerful and pleasant privilege of acceptance or rejection—mopping the bowl clean with a crust of "friendly" bread or slamming the silly book shut. We yet, *Deo Volente*, are granted certain powers and residual freedoms of choice.

It is sufficient, almost, that I say no more. I beg only that you allow me to note, with thanks and appreciation, that these essays came about as a result of the kind invitation of "Remi" Lacsamana, MD, who as Editor of the *Journal of the FMA* in 1989 invited me to write something of this sort. The ongoing support I received from Jacques Caldwell, MD, Dr. Lacsamana's successor, was equally gracious and supportive. I like to think that these accomplished physicians, both of them writers of happy merit, perceived with me that the practice of medicine, caught up to such a degree though it is in the success of its own technology, yet remains the most human and humane of endeavors. That they should have thought that I, an old-fashioned, solo, country, plastic surgeon, ensconced in a small bungalow surrounded by a live oak tree and a picket fence, could have something to say about the humanity and charm of what I get to do as a physician has done me great honor.

Most particularly, I wish to thank an eleventh man beyond the ten above: A. Bernard Ackerman, MD, veritably of New York, New York, who by some curious quirk or coincidence, or out of his own insatiably catholic curiosity and reading, stumbled on one of these essays, goodness knows where or how. Succor, as we all know, is properly predisposed to arrive at the penultimate eleventh hour. In this instance it was the eleventh man who strode onto my scene at what I shall also call the penultimate moment (and what "moment" may not be?) before the stroke of midnight . . . for I am well beyond high noon!

In any case, thus galloped into the complacency of my life the tall stranger, Dr. A., a gentleman-scholar-dermatopathologist (sic) who has been to Venice 29 (sic) times! Having found himself, by some peculiar means as I imagine it, stranded on a desert island between lectures and peregrinations to Venice and elsewhere, and with nothing whatsoever to read but an old copy of the *Journal of the Florida Medical Association*, he perforce read therein what I had written, requesting after his rescue that I send others of like ilk.

By this means I found myself caught up in the delightful current of his enthusiasm that these essays, so humbly written despite certain ostensible pretensions, might be worthy of a somewhat wider publication. While secretly thrilled, I naturally put on that trustworthy garb of modest diffidence, which he brushed aside, taking me off to dinner. I do thank him, not only for dinner, but beyond that for the warmth and generosity of his spirit, his hospitality, his example, and what has now become . . . how could it be otherwise given the above . . . his friendship.

He and I, as it turns out, have a similar taste in soup.

INTRODUCTION

About 15 years ago I started writing a diary. It was not because I thought I had anything to say to anyone, even myself, and certainly not to posterity.

Of course, one always dreams that one might be serendipitously "discovered" in some old moldering trunk 200 years from now by some old moldering scholar of that time who would immediately, recognizing the brilliance and worth of yourself, shout "Eureka" and forthwith publish your work by the Book-of-the-New-Millennium-Month-Club. Fondly one imagines historians of that new age, if it dawns, pouring over your every tidbit of syntax, discovering and debating over clues as to the reality of what I shall call life at the end of the twentieth century. I fantasize how my bones would rattle if someone would cry out "He is a Pepys newfound!," and that readers two centuries from now would be impressed and maybe even titillated by the intimacy of my disclosures, demonstrating among other things that I was a real man of my times, complete with a rather racy inner and, for that matter, outer life.

Contrary to Pepys, and to tell the truth too, we do not possess some lusty parlor-maid drifting about our house after whom I might hanker and slyly chase, even at the risk of a tongue lashing from my sweet wife and a slap on the face from the maid. If such delectations, however, did exist hereabouts, I am both too politically correct, and polite too, and in love with my wife three, to be remotely tempted. As well, I drink altogether too modestly, never having frightful binges and head-splitting hangovers to confess, preferring the olive in my martini and the shape of the glass to the gin within. I am invariably almost on time for work, and never more than two minutes late for the commencement of any surgery, which latter fact is the fault of traffic rather than myself. I am a "temperate" sort of man, in that sense rather like Professor Higgins, and lead a life where "hurricanes hardly happen," and rains in Spain never.

In a word, my circumstance is pretty prosy, replete with numerous insurance premiums to be paid and a considerable mortgage yet outstanding, despite the fact that everyone else my age is retired or almost. My diary is even worse than prosy: There is no chance that anyone will ever read it and say anything remotely like "Eureka!" It is a remarkable fact, I tell you right now, how pale, jejune, and picayune life on a day-to-day basis may be, even though as yet red blood may be coursing through your veins. Day in and day out you write the equivalent of "Dear Diary . . . I had a nice day today. The weather was good, but we need rain. One of the goldfish died, but it only cost 33 cents because I got three for a dollar. Well, that's about it. See you tomorrow!" Fifteen years of this, I tell you again, does not make a very good read.

No, I was clever enough to know that I was not writing a diary in order to record anything insightful or sanctimonious about my life, either per se or per posterity. Not at all! No, I decided I had better start a diary or else my life would be gone, and I would not have the least idea what had happened, and certainly no idea what the weather was on any particular day. It had become clear to me that I could not remember the least thing I might have done a mere two days past. To be so forgetful seemed to me terribly unfair to Life (with a capital L you notice) and which is granted us as an experience that after all is not necessarily a very common event in this universe. Yet here we are, somehow "chosen," granted this odd miracle which I, at least, was passing through as though I had supped daily on nothing more than lotus leaves and nepenthe. Surely, thought I, as a sentient creature, capable of questioning the stars and so on, I could at least do Life the honor of recording some something of its passage, even if I could not sing its praise with the eloquence it deserved.

I have never once looked back in my diary. The fond, if vague, hope that it might be useful as a means of searching out specific events, people, and places otherwise inaccessible to memory has been a hope dashed. It has no use except one, and that is, if I accidentally run across these stacks of paper, that they clearly demonstrate, to me at least, that I have lived, one day at a time. Although I never do, nor do I intend to, it is a comfort to me to know that at least for these past fifteen years I can, if called upon by some angel asking me precisely what I did on such and such a day, and what was the weather, and that my mortal soul depended on it, answer. Never mind that the answer is necessarily but the bare rattling bones of that day's doings, the subtle flesh long gone; I can, at least, contrive an answer. And every now and then, ever so slyly, and just to wake her up and provide a small modicum of entertainment, and to prevent her, my trusty amanuensis from becoming jaded with all the operation reports I have dictated to her, and which she has so faithfully transcribed over the years, I will throw in some ribald lusty tid-bit. Once, I recall, it had to do with the lush fantasy of dressing my wife in a Lady Hamilton costume, full of décolletage, and I in a Lord Nelson outfit, complete with a cocked hat and an eye patch (but both arms) just home from two years at sea, after defeating the French again, while Vesuvius smol-ders pregnantly in the background.

Now, indeed, that my wife has become my amanuensis I have gotten worse, and sometimes even dabble in X ratings. If only that moldy scholar might then by chance and fate be led, as to a needle in a haystack, to just there, they will see what a lusty lad I was after all, and damn the truth. I wonder if, in 2199, there will be a Book-of-the-Month-Club?

And so, as an offshoot to writing a personal journal vindicative of my fond hope in the possibility of reality's existence, and what was the weather, I conceived that the same could possibly be done for the ordinary, humdrum, everyday practice of medicine? We possess of medical writing so much that is so scholarly, so bright, so scientific, so terse, so timely, so well studied and researched by so many so learned in their fields. But what about people who are *not* particularly learned in their fields? What about those countless doctors, the vast majority indeed and myself among them, who day to day practice what they have learned, struggling to perfect it according to the mundane needs of their particular niche, and gradually, by slow trial and error, doing so. Prosaic though may be their concerns and their perceptions, might not these, too, be worth some slight recording? Is not the least most humble thing worth its small note in this big life?

Is this what I thought to record when Dr. Lacsamana asked me to write a monthly piece for the *Journal of the Florida Medical Association*? And so I commenced, never minding then or now if whatever I found to say held the least interest for anybody. I did it as I did my diary, in some large sense for myself, to discover, and maybe not to forget so quickly, what it was I was doing and maybe, just barely, thinking about. Whether these essays have any large relevance to medicine "as it is and was practiced in late 20th century America," I do not know; and scarcely care. They are a highly personal record, for which you must forgive me. The fact that they were written is some form of proof to myself that during the course of their writing I have been, at least, slightly alive. I feel most gratified with the hope.

And so we are going to drag these fellows out a little into the light of a wider world, allowing them to feel their way towards some definition of their own intent.

I wonder how it will turn out? Meantime I will carry on with my diary and who knows what I may discover beyond Lady Hamilton and his Lordship, if only my wife will put up with me! And if only I can live long enough! . . . which prompts me, as a physician, to suggest to you that you start your own diary young, stick with it, work through the weather, and ultimately you will, sooner than I, discover life to be more luscious than you might have thought!

There is no telling where one can lead oneself! I have no sooner finished the paragraphs above than, suddenly, full sprung, I see how lovely my wife would be as "Jane!" But myself ? Am I sufficiently advanced for a Tarzan outfit?

I quiver with possibility. There is no telling what my diary will divulge in the next fifteen years!

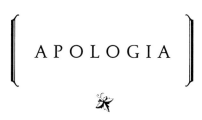

APOLOGIA

*Being in some considerable measure uncertain that anyone will be much
inclined to read any of what I shall call these "essays" I feel duty bound*
before they launch forth to introduce them, yet again, with a veritable
Apologia.

I rush to mention that I do not use the term "apologetically." My own fancy
(for I have not quite gone to the dictionary) tells me that an "Apology" and an
"Apologia" are two quite different things. I apologize for nothing, except perhaps my grammatical lapses and, even more tangentially, my devotion to the
parenthetical observation, which has always seemed to me more intriguing than
any thesis itself. Nor, by the way, do I wish in the least manner to diminish by
such rank "apologies" the faith that he who is "my publisher" has in the fact that
some handful of curious persons might wish to skim through an occasional of
these minor little *essais*. I might here add, parenthetically of course, that as their
author it would be my fond ideal if these essays could be read, so long as virtue
is not subverted, with a double martini at your side and a cat in your lap.

There is, after all, something to be said for the ambiance surrounding a
reader reading. I realize full well that there are those truly great readers who
in due course becoming great writers tell us how, for example, in the
trenches of World War I they carried some precious, battered volume of
Shakespeare, or maybe *The Faerie Queene*, and while being shelled took solace in the contemplation of beautiful words wonderfully writ. Most
recently in my own reading I note that George MacDonald Fraser, the cre-
ator of that sublime cad Flashman, tells us in his wonderful memoir *Quar-*

tered Safe Out Here of how he read *Henry V* while slapping mosquitoes in the midst of monsoons and dodging bullets when, at age 19, he was a part of the final drive to thrust the Japanese out of Burma.

But this is Shakespeare, who can lift at least some above mere bombardments and mosquitoes. As for Spenser, I confess that I am inclined to a greater skepticism, while admitting that our age, and I myself, are not so well inclined towards "fairy queens" as were those idealistic youths of World War I. Suffice it that some authors can rise above their readers' circumstance; and others not at all. We must, like certain restaurants, appeal to our clientele not through the meat of our intellect and argument but by means of the ambiance surrounding. The hope is, of course, that the flaws in the writing will be slyly mitigated by the comfort of the reader's circumstance, the crystal clarity of the martini to hand, the purring of the cat in your lap . . .

I beg you accordingly, if you really are going to read any of what I have written, to get comfortable!

Allow me, as well, this veritable Apologia, by which I mean more truly an explanation. "Explanation?" you may well ask? "Why should this essayist be allowed so much? Did Leigh Hunt feel obliged to write a tortuous preamble of 'Explanations' and 'Introductions' before launching any collection of his essays?"

I think not; and can only say that I, on the other hand, need must and, while thanking you for your generous indulgence, construe this need as being both rational and appropriate for two reasons.

The first states that possibly the most interesting thing about any essay is what is left out of it, namely why the essayist came to the topic at all? In this instance the essays which follow came about as the result of, first, a monthly deadline, and second, through my simple determination to select out of each month some highlight of my concern as it impinged on my rather small surgical practice. As a diary does for a day, I saw this as more or less an encapsulation of an issue-of-the-month. I decided, furthermore, that in this life there are things "Good" and "Bad" and of course if not downright "Ugly" why not "Homely," with its rich connotations of just "Down-Hominess" and trivia. As it turned out, the good and the bad and the homely often ran together. Even so I have attempted, for the reader's convenience and in retrospect, to separate these essays accordingly, thus breaking up the strict chronology of their writing. This was rather a difficult task, which I solved by placing a cat in my lap, and a martini at my side, and thus fortified skimmed through each of these, glancingly deciding to toss this or that into one category or the other. This took about half an hour, and if I apologize for anything it is that what purports to promise neat little categories of goodness, badness, and homeliness will prove to be rather more random. But that's life, isn't it?

Finally, I want to explain . . . and maybe just apologize a very little . . . that much in these essays is only topical to a moment now past. I think there are maybe too many perusals of the great silicone implant debacle, but this was, for a time, a most wretched concern, and its presentation by the media and the courts made many perfectly healthy ladies utterly ill with anxiety, if their silicone implants did not. There are numerous sidelong allusions to people and things, which only someone "inside" the medical profession, and at that in the state of Florida itself, might . . . or might not even then, come to think of it . . . appreciate or comprehend. Indeed, there may be so much of this sort of thing that as much as for any other reason I can quite fully understand how any reader of these words might quickly enough prefer just the martini and the cat, exclusive of the book . . .

For this reason, and because I thought it might be simple fun, and because I like a good footnote as much as a pair of parentheses, I have decided to include such asides and annotations, hoping that it will add a little interest . . . and ambiance, of course.

Is it not true, after all, that much of the practice of medicine and life itself, resides in the footnotes? One day, maybe, some brilliant someone (or is that what James Joyce already did in *Ulysses*?) will write a pleasant volume essentially of footnotes only, held together by just a very few words of text writ bold.

PREAMBULATION

Wherin I feel my way along toward a theme,
a voice, conceivably (even) some sort of meaning.

PREAMBULATION

In 1974 I arrived in Tallahassee, fully trained if by no means fully feath-
ered, to establish my practice in "Plastic and Reconstructive Surgery."
I brought with me all my worldly possessions, consisting mostly of old
books and an old cat packed into my relatively new Porsche 911. I rented a
little apartment in a big apartment complex almost generically identical to
the one I had lived in while doing my residency in Plastic Surgery at the
University of Florida, in Gainesville. I bought some pretty, if inexpensive,
furniture; and some beautiful silk flowers, playing it safe, which I stuck in a
vase. I carefully put my books in a bookcase, and so called it "home."

Within a few months my dear old friend, the cat, died. I bought a shovel,
and buried her beneath an azalea bush hard by the diminutive "patio" that
came with my apartment. I mourned her loss, but in due course other cats
came along, of equally delightful and I might even say "noble" character, as
you shall see; and dogs too, to be let in and out.

As for the Porsche, which for 5,000 borrowed dollars I had recklessly
purchased for morale purposes during the last year of my general surgery
residency at the Mary Hitchcock Memorial Hospital in Hanover, New
Hampshire, I ultimately gave it away to someone who could admire it more
than I. At the time I thought the gesture rather generous, but dare say you
will be inclined to join me now as I begin to reconsider it as simply foolish.
Although they never even saw the car, my two daughters irreverently berate
me for the brazen perfidy of the act, visualizing themselves at its wheel,
which I feel in turn grateful that they are not. In any case, I confess that even

at the time I gave it away there was behind that scene a sort of ulterior, squinty-eyed motivation, which consisted more of frustration and laziness than of generosity.

First of all, after the great oil embargo of 1973 when speed limits were so drastically lowered, I picked up a whole bunch of tickets with this Porsche, which scarcely knew how to drive under ninety. As I drove from New Hampshire down to Florida I found, by the way, Georgia particularly intolerant. Ultimately I had to take some kind of course, most offensive I thought to the dignity of my professional circumstance, or they might have thrown me into some kind of jail. Even a mere 25 years ago the times were simpler. In any case, I was granted back my license; but that terrible automobile had a mind of its own with which I was constantly wrestling.

Second, and even worse, this was a real Porsche, born of course in Germany and adapted to New England's climate, and without therefore any sort of air conditioning. Granted, the true aficionado scorns such conveniences in a Porsche as altogether demeaning to its engineering and performance, but in Florida an air conditioner in your automobile is perhaps slightly more desirable than the four wheels.

In any case, perhaps demonstrative of how few feathers I had as this fledgling whatnot-surgeon-though-I-was, having no knowledge of how to sell a car I found it much easier to give it away; and so did, essentially for the price of the recipient doing the necessary paperwork. Would, by the way, that the government and Health Care Industry might disencumber me so tolerantly of *their* paperwork in exchange for a Porsche; but never mind, perhaps I should be grateful that now, with a heavy sigh, those entities have taught me to fill in forms with my eyes closed, and sometimes maybe with my fingers crossed.

Suffice it that I bought a Toyota Celica, which did me quite well, and thank God was not performance oriented. I still drive it, maintaining at all costs its air conditioner, and thus have lived automotively happy ever since.

If, and for no other reason, I am faithful to this car it is because I have never, ever been given a ticket by it in, Lo!, these past 22 years. As well, it is embarrassing in its dilapidation (it has never been washed or seen the inside of a garage) in the eyes of our two daughters. They bitterly regret the Porsche-that-could-have-been-theirs, and are instead forced to blush whenever I have delivered them up to school in my Toyota, or even worse picked them up from some festive high-class affair where my car, and conceivably even myself, might actually be seen by their chic friends. All parents, as certainly you will acknowledge, have lurking beneath their superficial blandness a fierce little element of perversity, sometimes even passively aggressive.

In those days, plastic surgery, and "cosmetic surgery" even more, were scarcely known in Tallahassee. We are not the Florida of your dreams, or at least those depicted on the posters, which so suavely attempt to beguile northerners and even sophisticated Europeans to the pleasures of basking and balming. We remain a sort of outpost of the "Old South," and even the highway connecting us with Jacksonville and New Orleans had yet in those days great, unfinished gaps in it. We had essentially four restaurants, none of them of the "chain" variety so ubiquitous nowadays, the idea of dining out for fun having not quite yet dawned upon us. Our local medical society met monthly at Joe's Steak House, now long gone, and that was quite a sufficiency. The steaks were pretty good, and you got a choice of either sour cream or butter for your baked potato, so as a community of physicians we were quite content.

But it was this very sort of thing that so much charmed, not to forget the trees and Spanish Moss (*Tillandsia usneoides*) that so delight everyone who comes here. "Glooms of the live-oaks, beautiful-braided and woven . . . that myriad-cloven clamber the forks of the multiform boughs . . ." etc., as Sidney Lanier put it. There is in such images a rich suggestion of decadent possibility, which even if it turns out to be simply mildew nonetheless beguiles. I was immediately enchanted by the pleasant circumstance, almost palpably felt, of Tallahassee as an old southern town, but with the amenities of two excellent universities, a lovely unspoiled coastline 25 miles to the south, and an excellent hospital with a high-quality staff. It was a place neither then nor now very easy to get to, and so in its halfwise way stood apart, a little forgotten and remote in feeling. In this, and much else, it quite romanced my imagination.

Office space was at a premium. I ended up in a little cottage built in 1946, just a couple of blocks from the hospital, and used by a family practice physician until he retired just as I needed it. I was pleased by its good and homely atmosphere. In front there was a large live oak, which remains steadfast despite the ruthless incursions of road widening. Having a deeply ingrained need to surround property, like pictures, with some kind of frame, I had a pleasant, white picket fence placed about my periphery, and contrived to make a bit of a garden within. The waiting room, though small, I furnished as invitingly as I knew how, including a mess of plants, which we have ever since struggled to keep healthy and alive, remembering how I once read that you should be leery of going to doctors with dead plants hanging dolefully about the office. Because I was a veritable "Plastic Surgeon," I subscribed to a number of high-class magazines, for awhile going even so far as *Town and Country* and *The Magazine Antiques*, as I thought that these were doubtlessly what large-scale plastic surgeons in New York and maybe Los Angeles had scattered about their offices. It became our affirmed policy to give these away to individuals whenever they expressed an interest in them, thereby excusing them from the temptation to filch them, and by which means we avoided having two-year-old copies of *Field and Stream* equivalents lingering miserably about. On the walls I placed a number of nicely framed prints, some of which I tore out of an art book, showing mostly sailing scenes and Winslow Homer stuff, and which look (even yet!) quite attractive on the grass cloth walls we refurbished with. I got a very pretty oriental "runner" to go down the little hall, but this was finally dispensed with in a fine frenzy because, whenever your turned your back on it, it rushed over to cower against the southern baseboard, looking miserable. If anyone ever invents a way to truly keep a carpet from "creeping," he or she will instantly be made as rich as Croesus or the inventor of Velcro or the Hoola-Hoop.

We fitted up a couple of rooms for the purposes of consultation and examination, with skylights to let in the natural light, and created a fairly fully equipped operating room. I made a cozy office for myself, looking out over the trash cans of the chiropractor next door, but with the intervention of a few branches and leaves permiting me with relative ease to imagine it to be a woodland scene. It was rather like having a hotdog bun, nicely toasted, and filling it with large enough dollops of ketchup, relish, mustard and onions so that the dog itself is scarcely missed and easily imagined. It is always good to practice your imagination for healthy purposes, I think.

I bought an expensive ($600) reproduction Regency writing table for my desk, on which I have piled ever since books and papers, so the "Regency" part is quite obscured. In the kitchen we saw to it that there was a nice stock of junk food, with every now and then, consumed by a fine frenzy of guilt, some fruit. Off the kitchen is a small porch, embowered by overhanging trees, which actually are the chiropractor's, but which we get to enjoy more than he. I pictured, and indeed brought to pass for a period of time, light luncheons in that setting, surrounded by plants, let us say magnificently in bloom just for the record.

The neighborhood, although quite near the hospital, has become somewhat shabby since all the great practices moved out about the time I moved in, establishing themselves collegially in expensive, high-tech offices in a great "Medical Plaza" a mile from the hospital itself. I take, accordingly, a mild if somewhat contrary pride in being where I am. Happily we are next door to the chambers of our local medical society, staffed by an inimitable bunch of delightful people, who and which I like to think give us a certain cachet by proximity. Otherwise, we are surrounded by a nice selection of "alternative care" practitioners, including an acupuncturist and for a pretty period a real astrologer with suns and moons displayed. I welcomed the latter, for there is nothing wrong with having someone so conveniently close at hand in case of a particularly urgent need for specialized advice. A Rolfer came and went; but I never "Rolf."

In any case, never minding the astrologers and Rolfers, I determined to fight it out on this front, more or less steadfast in my determination to maintain what I shall hopefully call my ideals regarding the practice of medicine and surgery. Naturally one must be on guard, and I have faithfully kept my fingers crossed that the branches from the old oak tree, breaking off now and again, did not crash through our skylights or brain some one of my patients. The long-range goal, but one which did not dawn on me until ten years into my practice, was to fund the pension plan. By this time I was fifty, and it became clear even to myself, great giver-awayer of Porsches, that something of the sort should be in order. Like many others, doubtless, I often wished I had some huge inheritance to fall back upon; but in the event, as the Rubǎiyǎt said, what is wrong with a jug (or even a box) of wine, a loaf of bread, and Thou?

As for "Thou," this took the form of the wife of my dreams, who was willing to marry me in 1981, and regarding whom I need say no more here, for the gist of her meaning will become clear as these pages turn.

Of course I needed a bit of a staff. In those halcyon, pre-computer, pre-managed care, pre-pulse oximeter days, the physician-surgeon even so needed some assistance. I was told by a person of excellent authority that all that was necessary was "a 'girl,' a nurse, and a typewriter." The advice, which now smacks my ear as being pretty un-PC, was simplistic, but on the whole rather accurate. It was all, *pari passu,* that I knew to do in any event, and so I did just that.

Thus into this void came along (oh let me shower blessings upon her brow!) the delightful Miss Linda, age 20ish, who was immediately appointed "Office Manager." She remains to this day Office Manager, but is now grown to be the even more delightful Mrs. Linda Sipp, mother of two and wife of one, and possessed of the neat knack of growing better and more beautiful with every passing year. She came essentially, indeed, as a "girl," and now as a woman is not only beautiful and polished, but of such an astute and well-expressed intelligence that even strong men tremble before her quick perception and inquiring eye.

As for the nurse, she appeared as "Nurse Dee," who almost instantly charmed all patients and people with her mellifluous voice and gentle manner, and to such a degree that I believe they would sometimes come to me for their surgery just so they might be in her presence. Dee stayed with me for four or five years, and then ran off to marry an old-fashioned, southern, gentleman ophthalmologist, raising her family, and seen by me only in passing over the years. But now, most pleasant to note, with her family sufficiently grown, she has come back to the office, for yes we have grown a bit too, and needed an extra nurse. Who but she, if only she would; and she did.

As for the typewriter, it was an IBM Selectric, of course, which we thought terribly expensive. Having grown up toting around a Smith-Corona portable, with nary an electron to be seen anywhere hovering about it, I vaguely wondered why one needed these contraptions to be "Selectric," with all that concomitant expense?

I do not need to tell you how important the nurse is to any physician's practice, particularly a smallish, intimate one wherein the physician is struggling both to maintain his autonomy as a solo practitioner and, as well, to make ends meet. Nurse Dee got me off to a splendid start. But when she left we fell on slightly more difficult nursing times: A modest variety of nurses passed through our portals. For a few years we benefited from the presence of the rumbustious "Nurse Jane," who was wonderful too with people, and had a marvelous background by having for years scrubbed on every conceivable type of operation in the hospital. Jane would be perfectly capable of taking out your heart before lunch, dining, and putting it back in afterwards. She did a suction lipectomy on one of my love handles when we once had nothing better to do, and I wanted (a) to get rid of the love handle on that side,[1] and (b) to have the experience of the procedure at very low cost. Jane possessed a dauntless confidence, verve, and personality, and was one of those people everyone found grand fun to work with. But alas, her own heart, perhaps a little too dauntless, was lost to some *Don Giovanni* from a rough county adjacent to ours who played her music that was, sadly, not Mozart. Indeed, and no more need be said, rumor had it that he was not even in possession of a driver's license. He lured her into awkward moments and transactions, and she finally indeed had to flee our little coop, ending up in a less rough but more remote county in the farther west of our Panhandle. We mourned Jane, and what we considered her sad fate, and perforce struggled onwards.

Strangely, even so, over the years we somehow grew. We got another typewriter. In the early eighties, I bought the little cottage and made numerous additions and pleasant changes to it. We struggled with the garden, which is a bit too shady, being overhung to such an extent by our live oak. We became accredited as a Class II outpatient surgical facility. We necessarily had to buy an oximeter, and a wonderful gadget that has been too!

[1]My own experience is helpful in explaining just *why* suction lipectomy has assumed to itself such a place in cosmetic surgery. I have a small neck (15"), and so when I bought a shirt to fit my neck the midriff was invariably tight. Like just about anybody, I hated seeing the buttons taut over what I shall call my belly, even on occasion to a point where a little peek-a-boo flesh was seen. No one wants to go to a plastic surgeon who is so displayed! Accordingly, the moment opportune due to a cancellation of something or other, I threw some Xylocaine about in one of my love handles, and we made a small incision, introduced the cannula, turned on the machine, and in a jiffy I was reduced. Well, even Jane got a little scared, and stayed in one place a bit too long; so I now have a bit of a groove, too, on that side. But she got out enough so that never again have my shirts been tight. If I am slightly asymmetrical, not having "done" the other side, I consider it but the asymmetry of "art," and in any case, my problem solved, I am a happy patient. My wife is fine with my asymmetry too, and I even flatter myself with the sanguine hope that she may find it interesting.

We were sold a terrible computer system; struggled with it and, not being able to give it away, tossed it and bought another one. We needed a bit more staff. We flourished, at least in happiness in the work place, and paid our bills. There was a year or two when we were unable to fund our pension plan, but for the most part once we got it going we contrived to do so within reason.

My big regret has been that we never could have an office cat. OSHA, a post-modern ombudsocracy, would have surely tortured us. But how can you be truly "Homely" if you do not have a cat? And yet even I knew we could not afford one, malpractice being what it is, and never minding that we would not want to cause someone's allergies to flare up. Cats have, after all, been seriously shown to raise the liability stakes.

I am quite serious indeed. Years ago, I confess with a decent modicum of pleasure too, I recall reading of an "incident" highly reported in a south Florida newspaper about a surgeon who, following "office surgery," had offended the patient by placing a black cat on her "tummy." Although I would like to have a black cat, the maneuver at that time seemed to me altogether interesting and curious. Of course there was some awful suit, but surely more would be required than merely placing a black cat on a tummy, and so it proved. The more proximate, as I think they call it, cause was some slight misplacement of the belly button. The combination of a belly button not quite where it should be with a black cat suddenly appearing on site clearly became sufficient cause for litigation. I have no idea how it all turned out.

I have since thought it rather unfair, nonetheless, having accidentally on rare occasions ever so slightly misplaced a belly button or two myself. It has seemed to me, on the other hand, that the placing of a gentle, soft, neutered, declawed, purring cat on a patient immediately after surgery might, on certain, specific occasions, the details having clearly been discussed and spelled out beforehand, prove highly soothing. But the cautionary tale above noted has probably saved me from succumbing to such temptation.

But one of these days, if I ever retire, perhaps just once . . . perhaps as my ultimate surgical act, longing to give it a go myself . . . I might bring our sweet Pussy Willow to the office and place her on some postoperative "tummy," the dressing, of course, fully in place and a nice soft blanket overlying. Despite the risk of litigation I would simply like to see what, indeed, would happen.

Might not I, after all, at least once in my career, try living a little dangerously too?

Beyond which I will nevertheless be extra careful exactly where I put the belly button.

THE
GOOD

INTRODUCTORY: THE GOOD

I do not think I learned it in kindergarten, where some would have it that we learned "All We Know," but it may not have been many years after that I was struck with the peculiar word printed on light bulbs, "Mazda." It was too strange a word to warrant neglect. And then, surely not too long afterwards, I became aware of Ahriman, the spirit of darkness against which we contend and, to our great relief at age eight when we push on the light switch, conquer. I dare say I became a Manichean by the time I was in the eighth grade.

Unless I have had a martini, I never lecture my friends on the struggle between Light and Dark, because I think most of us take for granted that it is pretty closely balanced. It is very hard for me, as I glance about this mortal coil, not to believe that there is a remarkable poise between Good and Evil, Light and Dark, and the struggle between them, so relentless that to think there is a clear predominance of one over the other is a bit absurd. Of course, I am a bit absurd, too; but, on the other hand, I would in my absurdity defy anyone to prove to me that there is other in this world than a rather interesting contention going on between Good and Bad. I leave out for the moment mere Homely, which, though apparently a simple featherweight, may yet slyly, but perhaps in the final analysis, tip the scales one way or the other, after all!

In any case, and to put it in homely terms indeed, I have comforted myself with the belief that we, by which I include regular folks like you, and me, and the rest of the universe, are nothing but a great, grand experiment in God's test tube. I perceive this "God" a little after the fashion of the 18th century Rationalists, or maybe a little like those "drowsy" Beings of Conrad Aiken's who lean "immeasurable as clouds, above a chess-board world." I see the experiment as beyond all doubt the most fascinating that a universe, or the God running it, might contrive: namely to mix into some primordial soup an absolutely equivalent amount of Black and White, Good and Bad, and then throw into it an interesting catalyst, which is ourselves. This catalyst would stand precisely halfway between Good and Bad, the angels and the brutes of Pascal, and be endowed with Free Will. Given this ultimate attribute, denied rocks and clods, what effect would it have on the balance between Good and Bad as it chose between them, perhaps now tending towards the one and then again towards the other? Would Good win out, and the universe blossom in ways beyond imagining; or would Bad, causing a laboratory explosion, end with a Bang the experiment? What small decision, what tiny exercise of a bit of Free Will might make the difference one way or the other?

In a confusing universe, where sometimes you can hardly know this from that, we make our choices, hoping that they will be good enough to beat back the weight of Bad. The physician is continually faced with these decisions like everyone else, and, yes, even the plastic surgeon if you will allow me. We plastic surgeons deal, after all, in the dissolution of the body, too, which can have as a side effect depressing repercussions on the mind and spirit. We also attempt (as is our oath!) to maintain the Good of Health and Well Being as do other real physicians. Indeed, not to be overly presumptuous, the plastic surgeon attempts to "uplift" even beyond health, that baseline which, in sickness, the patient so yearns once more to achieve, by decisions rightly made which will gain for even the healthy something in fact better than their former selves. I beg you not to argue with me too overly on this point, for I have seen too often these positive benefits: the enhancement of the person's whole perception of themselves, and a happier harmonization of that dainty balance between mind, body, and spirit.

But, as Hippocrates so nicely put it in the paraphrase I often repeat to myself, "Art is long, Life is short, Judgment difficult, the Moment fleeting, the Outcome uncertain, ..." Our free will, and our best judgments, must be exercised frequently enough within the dubious circumstance of mists and shapes but dimly seen. We squint into the mystery that is within us and around us, and make our choice, hoping it is good.

Thus I have squinted at these essays. They are all Homely, whether "Good" or "Bad," but these I have chosen to place in the category of Good have been so placed out of my own hopeful perception that somewhere in each of them is lodged a happy possibility, a something that seems good, and if elaborated upon might become more so beyond its immediate implications. What I have seen in them of Good another might not find. But anyway, the number of these Goods outweighs the number of those I determined would stand for Bad, which may suggest to you my own bias respecting the outcome of that struggle between Light and Dark, and our part in it. Nor will I let you forget Homely either: A wild card in this equation, but which might make as curious a difference as, for example, made that least quantum or quark at the beginning of time which, if there had been one more or one less we are told, would have created a universe altogether different, and inconceivably beyond our capability to imagine. I, for one, would like to see more articles in medical journals on the subject "Chaos in Medicine."

Of course I do not mean the simple, ordinary, everyday, lower case "c" chaos that involves running an office, seeing patients, and keeping the plants alive. I mean real Chaos, of the kind that happens with ventricular fibrillation and looking under a teenager's bed or, more happily, the Chaos that postulates (has this become a cliché yet?) that the flapping of a butterfly's wing in the Himalayas can be directly responsible for a tornado in Iowa. I am thrilled with the theory that these extraordinarily disparate events, so seemingly arbitrary, should be behind the scene so interconnected. Suddenly, and as by magic, so much that has seemed hectic, haphazard, exhausting, meaningless, and depressingly existential now becomes endowed with a significance of comprehensive proportions.

I saw a TV program on Chaos a number of months ago, and more recently have read half a book on it, so I know what I am talking about. But it was not until reading about iteration that I began to see the bright light of its full meaning. I don't think I have ever said this word "iteration" aloud, but mean pretty soon now to unleash it amongst my closer acquaintances and see how they bear up. Having one adolescent daughter and another who thinks she is already 13, I have necessarily had a good deal of experience with the iterative process, as has any parent who has had to say things over, and over, and over again, into mostly deaf ears. Quite naturally, such an experience gives this word a bad name, endowing it with an implied frustration, and even a kind of simple despair. But Iteration, the Grand Iteration of Chaos Theory, is on the other hand mood elevating, implicit with high hope, and giving of credibility even to that least Biblical sparrow who falls, and is marked and magnified by the iterative equation no less than the beat of the butterfly wing.

Indeed, in the book on Chaos that I have halfway read, even that least known fragment of energy, the quantum, gets itself endowed with a capacity to have changed the shape of our universe. Now it seems pretty nifty to me that the quantum, that very least bit of anything, could have such a profound significance on the meaning of the whole. For those of us who would like to have our simple faith buttressed by rational argument, here, clearly, is something to grasp at, harboring within itself a significance that we are by no means mere motes in a vast universe, drifting senselessly about. I do not mean, you understand, to sound like Wartly Bigsly, that interesting toad in the *Archie and Mehitabel* essays, who sat complacent beneath a mushroom, thoroughly determined he was the center of all about him. But still, it is rather nice to believe, even if we do not have pretty wings, that perhaps by flapping our arms we can play a potent role in the appearance of a rainbow on some planet circling Alpha Centauri. This is heady stuff. But if the Himalayan butterfly can pull it off, why not we as well?

But never mind all this enhancement of our own cosmological significance. Getting down to the sterner nitty-gritty of everyday medical practice, I am thankful to have been given a theory on which I can hang my cosmological hat, and better comprehend the curious chaos which whirls about me. What least thing that we do for a patient does not have its profound effects in some astonishing distant arena? Conversely, what least outward gesture might prove the preliminary tremor of an ultimate earthquake off the Richter Scale? You know the scenario: a little bleeding here, a bit of emesis there, and suddenly a procedure perfectly organized as though from a textbook flies into disarray; blood and guts are all over the floor, and you may even have to call a pathologist, or, God help us, a lawyer.

These disasters all have something to do with a torus which, as all torus-lovers know, looks something like a doughnut somehow, or otherwise may slyly resemble a folded piece of paper, the fold representing the area of (nice phrase) "cusp catastrophe." In any case, disaster and catastrophe have about them some kind of funny edge, which one can quite abruptly, just as Columbus' sailors thought they would, fall over to find oneself suddenly in a world of monsters, and/or (in our case) litigation, i.e., Chaos. The awful offal hits the fan, so to speak.

What an edge this is! My own most striking memory of a "catastrophe cusp" derives from medical school. I was on my surgery rotation and, of course, holding the retractor (and feeling quite giddy to start with) when the Great Surgeon decided, as a sort of afterthought at the end of doing something or other to a bile duct, to do a quick needle biopsy of the pancreas prior to closing. He was a very clever surgeon and had already asked me a bunch of questions during the procedure about which I knew little, being after all just the poor medical student. I was hanging from the retractor on the veritable edge of a torus myself, trying not to look pale and syncopal. He stuck the needle into the pancreatic unknown, and the room immediately filled with blood. Everyone went over the edge. It proved, later of course, to be a classic case, as has been famously called, of "nicking the aorta." In retrospect, I find comfort in the knowledge that this was nothing but an example of that interesting and infinitely fine margin between chaos and order. It was probably merely related to someone on a planet circling Alpha Centauri flapping his wings, or arms, or whatever, that morning.

So, even though one can take comfort in this theory, which gives us back maybe some of the meaning taken away by those villains Copernicus, Darwin, Marx, and Freud, with this knowledge comes also a real burden of responsibility. We now need to be even more thoughtful about what we do, because the effects can be so profound, not only here but even wherever in a far-distant space-time dimension. But isn't it good to know, after all, that we are all one, a happy, "happy few, we band of brothers," as Shakespeare, Kenneth Branagh, and Laurence Olivier have all said, all of us wonderfully interrelated in a forever dimension, making the universe go round?

Perhaps I'll even read the last half of that book, although just the first seems quite enough.

"PRACTICING" MEDICINE: I.

As is my wont, I found myself the other day wrestling with a breast. Before anyone jumps to lurid conclusions, let me hasten to add that this was nothing less than a highly professional enterprise. Even cardiologists may remotely know that this is the sort of thing, after all, that plastic surgeons "do." Though it may not seem a particularly subtle exercise to those of you more intimately involved with, for example, the Foramen of Morgagni[1] it is nevertheless a more delicate undertaking than might meet the wide eye of the casual student of the swimming suit edition of *Sports Illustrated*.

After all, the effects of the breast's contour on mankind have been arguably as profound, perhaps more so, than those of its otherwise "simple" function as a pleasant gland delivering mother's milk on occasion. This may, of course, be a moot point, and I would certainly not wish to disparage the mammary gland as being in its functional capacity secondary to its curious power as an aesthetic "shape." But how many other organs were inspiration in the design of the champagne glass (not the flutey kind, of course)?

What I mean is that this is a serious subject, capable of exciting strong emotion in the population at large, and lawsuits for the plastic surgeon in particular.

[1] Giovanni Battista Morgagni, 1682–1771 who through his great work *De Sedibus . . . The Seats and Causes of Disease* brought medical practice into the modern world by noting that sickness arose from the disease affecting individual organs rather than as a result of vague "humoral imbalances," and that symptoms were "the cry of the suffering organs." An anatomist essentially, his name is attached to many bits of anatomy, the above mentioned "Foramen" being a weak space in the diaphragm, beneath the sternum, where a hernia can occur.

But enough of apologia. These breasts against which I was contending my steely nerves had nursed a few children and, to boot, had about them a treacherous asymmetry. There was simply a built-in nonaesthetic bulge recalcitrant to all my, what shall I call it?, "art." I never got it quite the way I wanted it, but nonetheless it was enough better so that I elected to go with what seemed possible, accepting the fact that I might have to do what we euphemistically call a "touch-up" (no charge to the patient) at some later moment of enlightenment.

As I was doing this operation, I thought to myself how this was indeed "practicing" surgery, and that after all these years (and I'm not so bad at this operation) I found myself curiously perplexed. I took comfort in the knowledge, chaos aside, that physicians of all ilks occasionally find themselves a bit bothered and bewildered. The only way to overcome such dilemmas is to "practice" your way out of them. It can be a lonely moment. The hideous shadow of perceived ineptitude asserts its baleful influence, subverting even the confidence of The Great Surgeon (maybe). Learning to deal with such subversions is a part of what we describe as "the practice of medicine."

My most memorable experience of this sort, beside which this resistant mastopexy pales by contrast, occurred in 1967. Having survived a classic (every other night on call at the hospital) rotating internship, I spent three delightful years on the south coast of Newfoundland as a district medical officer. I forgot everything I had been taught, but learned how to pull teeth without breaking most of them off. With this background I went off to Africa for a year as the solitary physician to a mission hospital run by Austrian nuns in Malawi. They hailed me, generous spirited creatures that they were, as a marvel sent from heaven, and I did my level best to act like what they wanted me to be, casually sprinkling my conversation with schistosomes and hoping they would provide me a tooth to pull.

Instead, I was presented with a young girl possessing a hemoglobin well below five, and an abdomen so appallingly distended that I was fearful we might all blow up if I tapped on it whatsoever. By way of temporizing I called

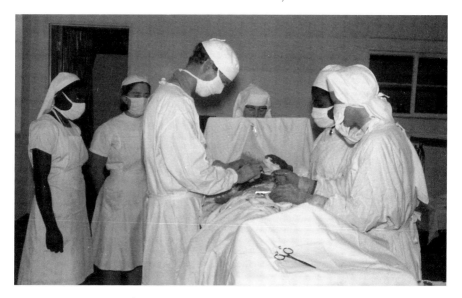

Trying hard not to faint while doing a little surgery at the Mission Hospital, Mamitete, Malawi, Africa. Note the total absence of an IV drip.

on Science, and begged the Sisters to unlimber the antique x-ray machine (to them an irrelevant accessory) which even unplugged looked vaguely lethal. We contrived a picture that showed nothing but emptiness. By this time I had read in my pocket Manson[2] that Africans had a higher incidence of volvulus than other folks, and armed by this slender fact closed my eyes to all else and exclaimed, "It's a volvulus; we have to operate!"

I raced for a surgical text and found nothing but huge, moldering German tomes, all in Gothic script. I looked at such pictures as I could discover but, of course, there was no hint to be gained.

When I made the incision, the patient's intestines seemed to fill the room, floating out every which where. My own blood volume, on the other hand, sank below my knees and I came exquisitely close to fainting.

[2]Sir Patrick Manson, 1844–1922, or, as he was termed by 1913, "The Father of Tropical Medicine," notable for his discovery that the filaria was transmitted to humans by way of the mosquito, thus paving the way for the discovery of the mechanism by which malaria is carried.

The ether dripped onto the mask, the sun dropped red in the ominous west, and I knew I had to attempt something before the monsoon was upon us. I muttered words to the effect that this operation required serious thought and marched about the white-walled room ostensibly "thinking," but more truly just managing to pump a little blood up to my Circle of Willis.[3] To make a longish story shorter, I made a lot of little enterostomies, bit by bit somewhat deflating these monstrous bowels, gently twisting this way and that in the hope that some marvelous unwinding would occur. It did not but, at least, I finally got everything back in, contriving as I backed out a little red-rubber-tube jejunostomy. I did not believe she would survive.

For me this experience has always defined at its most basic level "the practice of medicine/surgery." Even if I had had, in clear English, a copy of Cecil and Loeb,[4] I would have come just as close to fainting because C and L, etc., only tell you about blood pressure, in itself doing nothing to keep it up. Even HCFA[5] guidelines would not have helped had they existed! I was it, alone, with only my brains, bones, and autonomic nervous system, not to forget the Foramen of Morgagni.

We physicians are the vehicles through which the abstract theories and general knowledge of health and disease are translated into specific action. Try as it will, even the government will never quite succeed in substituting data for a doctor.

---

[3] Named for Thomas Willis, 1621–1675, who described this "circle" formed by blood vessels coming from the front of the brain and the back, located at the brain's base in rather difficult and awkward fashion. It is very nice to have blood going through these conduits, and let us hope the poor brain itself under the circumstances described.

[4] A voluminous textbook, famous for even more than its volume, which more or less covers all diseases, but not necessarily answering the physician's every question by any means whatsoever.

[5] HCFA: A jolly governmental bureauocracy which quite properly stands for "Health Care Finance Administration."

Well, the breast did well enough and had no complications. The patient is quite content actually, but I am glad to say is going to let me do just a teeny "touch-up" in due course nonetheless.

As for the African girl, the next morning, lo!, her tummy was flat and she was eating nsima, "grits" to us in the south. I took the tube out after a few days and she went home.

In her case, of course, the Sisters had said some nice prayers that first night and, as you know, there is nothing wrong with that either in "the practice of medicine."

"PRACTICING" MEDICINE: II. KEEPING YOUR FINGERS IN THE PROPER ORDER

A trouble with scientific papers is that they are divorced almost entirely from the niggle-naggle of medical practice. And everyone knows it's the niggle-naggle that drives one mad, and can get you into trouble as well.

I am sure you have read those articles that describe how to deal with, for example, awful complications. They are often gathered into the dispassionate embrace of "The Great Medical Center," which culls them preferably from someplace "Elsewhere" than themselves. These sometimes devastating horrors are reported with the same scientific detachment one might apply to observations of an ant farm, or a tadpole losing its tail. If such complications had happened in my practice, I would, myself, be wringing my hands and racing to the *Oxford Dictionary of Synonyms of Emotional Comfort*, if it existed, to ply my patient with.

Scientific-article-patients, on the other hand, seem to accept the worst with wonderful equanimity, and are gracefully prepared to go through innumerable further procedures and miseries to be finally restored to some vague semblance of their former selves. They do not appear tempted ever to litigate (wretched word!). Perhaps by getting "their" complication into medical print they are content with that as a sufficient solace.

These niggling aspects of medical practice are given short shrift by science. Yet when you get right down to it this aspect of our professional life is surely the most demanding feature of what we do, particularly in an age when all manner of people in three-piece suits are waiting to wring us dry of our last drop of ectoplasm.

Clearly, "practicing" medicine is to some significant degree the art of telling people what we cannot accomplish. This greater or lesser fragment of information must be conveyed without undermining either our integrity or the confidence we would like the patient to feel toward our efforts. We tell folks that this or that drug or procedure is fraught with hideous complications, including Death, Destruction, and Leukopenia, and in the same breath (smile) suggest that everything will after all be quite all right. We then proceed, hoping that the aforementioned "D, D, and L" do not occur to someone who might possibly be made a little angry over it.

I think I am having these thoughts because I think that lately I have had a rash of people who have seemed more than usually disappointed about certain results of my "art." (Never mind that in the augmentation mammoplasty business everyone wants to be bigger.) Perhaps I am losing touch a little with how to go about certain of even my most familiar procedures. I guess this can happen, for old ways of doing things, good though they may be, are necessarily and insidiously displaced by new approaches interjecting themselves between the lines of old habits. Despite what you read and hear at seminars, these interjections do not always quite work out as beautifully as the article or seminar suggested. So all of us keep "practicing."

Some people, of course, learn things more quickly than others. Everyone's capability to learn and adjust has what I shall call its own cybernetic algorithm, and I think that, even if memory is less with age, the algorithm may be better because of experience.

It is this thesis that I am attempting to explore, and with luck may even prove at least to myself, by teaching myself (yes, at this tender age) how to play the piano. This was no mean decision. I have been taught since a tiny tot to understand that I have absolutely no ear for music whatsoever. In the second grade, at a Christmas choir in which the whole school participated, I was weeded out amongst a hundred little voices and cast forth for the awkward sound I was making. I can remember the moment to this day: The

choir director heard something "wrong" way up in the upper left hand corner. The upper left hand corner sang. It was somewhere in the top row of
the upper left hand corner. The top row sang. "There it is," he said, the "it"
being me. I was quietly excised, while all the other little kids, thrilled that
they weren't "it," watched me remove myself.

But over the years it has come very slowly to my comprehension that just
perhaps this whole episode was a tremendous error, that the horrible sound
was from the little boy next to me, and that I might, after all, be better than
"they" ever thought.

At least, thought I, now I can bring some intellect of a sort to it. So I got
books and have been plinking away, late at night or in other nondescript
hours when no one was around who might sue. (After all, how much can
anyone bear of things like "Home on the Range"?) Well, I finally have
achieved a few pieces I can actually play: one of the simplest tunes probably
ever written by Beethoven in his sleep, and a "Twinkle Twinkle" variation by
Wolfgang Amadeus Mozart, who was not, I am told, poisoned by Salieri.

I am going about this learning exercise rather like a parrot speaking
words, but hoping unlike the parrot that comprehension will somewhat follow, maybe a little bit. The sounds come forth, and this is sufficient delight.
Yet, even in the midst of thinking that I have achieved some beautiful bit,
suddenly one finger will go wrong and all the others tumble after. Helpless,
I have to start over from the beginning. I am told that this is bad by people
who know, and maybe I will even grow out of it, but it is interesting to me
how the error of just one finger causes all the others to fumble in disarray,
the whole mess of fingers collapsing like dominos.

I don't think a lot has been written about how to think about practicing
music or medicine. There are a lot of awfully good general principles, which
may be more or less complicated in their enumeration by various authors,
from Hippocrates to Osler, and all of us in the final analysis develop our own
methods. One of the most delightfully conceptualized, within my own spe-

cialty, is that by Dr. D. Ralph Millard in his *Principlization of Plastic Surgery*. A great innovator, and with a style altogether unique within the framework of medical writing, Dr. Millard thoughtfully accompanies his beautiful volume with a blue bookmark on which are printed, in gold, 33 "Great Points" that summarize the percipient qualities brought into play by the thoughtful practitioner of medicine and surgery. These range from considerations of "No Harm," "Patient Desires," "Literature," "Record," "Robin Hood" (you have to read the book), "Graft," "Flexibility," and "Go for Broke." Although I respect every one of his observations, and try to keep them in mind more or less most of the time, 33 is a hard list to remember if you misplace the bookmark.

My own "great rules for the practice of medicine" are accordingly more general, and because I get to write this essay, I can foist them on you, if only as curiosities:

1. Everything will be all right. (Believe this!)
2. If the patient walked into the hospital, it is desirable that he/she also be able to walk out.
3. Keep it simple. (Don't needle biopsy around in the pancreas as an afterthought to the main procedure.)
4. Remember that everyone would prefer not to have to come to you no matter what your brilliance, competence, or charm, and treat them accordingly.

Of course I could go on but pretty soon I would have 33 points myself and would have to publish a bookmark at doubtless my own expense.

You can trust your own 33 points anyway. Just make sure you don't ever leave one out, even accidentally, when treating your patients. It will come back to haunt you.

And keep your fingers in proper order, of course.

WHALES,
MAYBE CODFISH

After 25 years away from my merry and memorable years of practice on the south coast of Newfoundland, I recently made a "sentimental journey" back to Hermitage Bay and the little town of Hermitage where I practiced as the District Medical Officer. From this locale I served the medical needs of approximately 14 small villages scattered up and down that rough and beautiful coast from a 40-foot boat, dispensing medicines and pulling teeth as the need required. (There was certainly no dentist within a few hundred miles.)

Let me spare you the sentiment. Suffice it to say that on my return I met many old friends, all of whom looked not a day older than I remembered them, and all of whom said I looked not a day older than they remembered me, which shows you how kind memory is in the final analysis.

I was amazed by the changes that had occurred. When I lived there, the only means of communication was by boat and telegraph over some sort of precarious wire I suppose. I would get telegrams from little outport villages, cryptic messages stating, "Doctor, come quick, baby won't come." Off I would rush into the night and weather, chugging along at some five knots over sometimes turbulent seas, usually to find the baby had after all come along quite well and was now squalling in its crib. Thank God it was, because, to tell the truth, I scarcely know what I would have done had there been any particularly real emergency.

As for electricity, this was available to a very few of the "privileged," such as the "town merchant" (his merchandise might fill an area 8' x 8'),

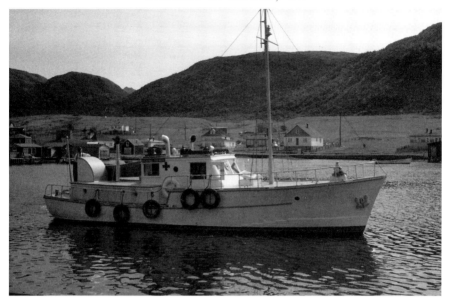

"The Doctor's Boat." I am lurking within.

the Anglican rector in Pushthrough, and of course my own, the doctor's house. There were two automobiles on the Peninsula, which were brought over by boat, connecting two of my villages by a precarious road across a bog, through valleys flanked by towering rock and lowering moor, with everywhere the distant view of a gorgeous ocean when the fog did not occlude it.

It was a wonderful almost-three years, but by the time I left I could hardly pronounce medical terms, having, rather like Robinson Crusoe, forgotten the language. The laboratory tests I had available consisted of an old optical hemoglobinometer. To whom, except to another physician, do you speak such a word? Like Crusoe I did not practice medical terms out loud to the rocks and wind. Indeed, I ultimately had to leave or I would never have been able to return to the so-called "mainstream" of medicine and residency without going through medical school all over again.

There is now a road that drops down from the Trans-Canada Highway some 250 miles to Hermitage. For tradition's sake, it seemed intolerable to my sensibilities to arrive by that road. Accordingly my wife, our nine-year-old daughter, and I took the "new" coastal boat, rushing along at 21 knots. We sailed into a scattering of the villages that still remain, these now numbering, as a result of government centralization policies, only a fraction of what once existed.

We were lucky. The weather could not have been better for us, with just a touch of fog here and there, lifting to show the sun bursting through white and blue cascades of sky above rocky cliffs and promontories dropping sharply into the sea . . . all comfortingly unchanged.

But that was all that was unchanged. Hermitage now comes complete with a plethora of traffic and automobiles including street signs and stop signs. A satellite dish has brought TV and American soap operas to the people. All the cars are shiny new. The old four-square houses, painted various rather crazy colors, have been replaced by neat new white one-story bungalows with all the amenities, including central heating. The only thing that hadn't quite made it to Hermitage was "la nouvelle cuisine," because the dinners we were invited to remained classically boiled, with rutabagas, turnips, potatoes, carrots, and codfish still dietary staples. Well . . . , you can't have everything all at once, can you?

Of the above, it's about codfish that I would like to write. For some reason, despite the rather tortuous analogy, I want to relate the postmodern physician with what has occurred to the codfish off the coast of Newfoundland, most particularly the Grand Banks.

Maybe I need not write more if I say, in a simple phrase, that both the cod and the physician have in their identities been raped and pillaged by bureaucrats who, in essence, can scarcely tell a codfish from an MD. Our identity and meaning have been torn from us. We have all been left either drowning (if you are a physician) or gasping (if you are a codfish) in the air, beating our tails and fins in some pathetic convulsion as we see ourselves slaughtered.

Because of government policies, bureaucratic interference, and the perception of the codfish as little more than an inanimate rock, a kind of fodder of the sea as opposed to a living, miraculous resource that it once was, the fishery is essentially dead. The fishermen are all going on welfare and are being paid not to fish, at least for the moment. Their rugged, stern independence; their tremendous ability over the past 300 years to survive and make do for themselves on a rough coast, have been torn from them, and within less than a generation a welfare mentality is being created.

So also have government, the law, and the media torn from the physician our meaning, our professional status, our role respectfully perceived as healers, capable of hard work and of trust. We too are little more than fodder in a sea of bureaucrats, whose bottom-line concerns relate to economics and ego, with no more conception for the physician's professional ideals than those other egos who so readily slaughter fish or forest.

What I saw in Newfoundland angered me. The cod are gone. The people have become enmeshed in the web of welfare statism. The physician, in a curious fashion, seems to me similarly threatened by a kind of extinction. We are similarly enmeshed. One is tempted to despair just a bit.

But then I think of that coast, its rocks, its sky, its fog, and those seas which yet may be capable of rebirth. In the mid-1960s, when I was there, cod were still plentiful, but there were no whales. The Norwegians had slaughtered them ruthlessly, even down to the smaller ones. When it became economically unprofitable they finally left off. But on this trip, I saw, as we went along by the coastal boat, innumerable whales, the plumes of their breathing catching the light as they blew, moving as gracefully as ballet dancers despite their mass. Sometimes we could hear their exhalations, even over the noise of the diesels. What a hope this seemed to me.

Maybe the codfish, now that no one is fishing for them because there are so few, will come back. Maybe some sort of enlightenment will dawn on bureaucrats and legislators. Or maybe, if it doesn't dawn, this breed will die off and more enlightened leaders will see that codfish and physicians alike are indeed a resource, to be trusted, to be valued, a part of nature to be used wisely.

Yes, I was glad to see that the shape of the hills was just the same as it always was and the sky still as beautiful a cobalt blue.

And the whales were back. It brings tears to one's eyes, if you will allow the final sentiment.

Might not the cod replenish as the whales have started to do, and the Grand Banks be restored as one of the world's wonders?

And why not, even, as a trusted resource the physician?

LI'L MIRACLE SOCKER

I wish to sing both the praises and the subtle pitfalls of "not thinking." Not being a psychiatrist, nor even a "Pop" psychologist, unless being a plastic surgeon qualifies, I grant myself accordingly all the authority that ignorance permits to discuss this subject.

I know, of course, there is this somewhat technical thing called Denial, which addresses people who block out all manner of discomforts thereby permitting them to carry on or, at least, creep on through life. It is not about this grand sort of Denial that I write, but rather the helpful distinction between that mere psychiatric diagnosis and the more pervasive value of just "not thinking."

With Denial something is blotted out. You don't even know you're blotting it out, and you go around looking glassy eyed and vague. When people, for example, ask where your hideous scars came from after you had been gnawed on by an alligator and you say, "What scars? What alligator?," I think you are practicing Denial. Such a flagrant rejection of reality is not what I mean. I have in mind the far more useful, conscious willingness to suppress thinking, so you can better enjoy lunch instead.

My own mind seems to me to go about suppressing almost everything within it almost all the time. As illustration, I offer those occasional moments when images well up before me of past misdeeds and *faux pas*: I cringe remembering when, having just met a young man at a moment in my own youth when I greatly admired the poetry of Dylan Thomas, I thought I was paying him a compliment by haplessly blurting out how remarkably his physiognomy resembled that of the poet's. The remark was the end of the beginning of any hope of friendship whatsoever.

Then there was the awkward time when, in some posh Park Avenue apartment at a dinner party where I was trying to wow the young lady who had complimented me by the invitation, I was served a large, round, green, head (it seemed to me) of lettuce with some orange lubricious soup on it reminiscent of Russian dressing. As I cut into it, it flew off my plate and rolled across the green Aubusson carpet leaving, to everyone's horror and not least my own, a trail of dressing.

Then there was the time as a young ensign on the bridge of a great air-craft carrier leading the fleet through the Mediterranean, the admiral ordered me to the radio to say something like "Fleet maneuver, 20 degrees left rudder to course blah-blah." On the end of the "blah-blah" I thought it would be nice to add "please." I was nearly forced to walk the plank, and as you see never made the Navy my career. I suppose we all have a dozen, or a dozen thousand, of these little memories just below the surface that strug-gle continually to well up at curious moments.

As an aside, surely the effort to suppress such trivia is one of the reasons people like eating so much because food, and junk food particularly, is a strong adjunctive measure toward effective mental suppression. There is simply nothing like a bag of "snuck" potato chips. If you happen to have some beluga caviar on a nice crust with a squeeze of lemon juice and a tiny dollop of Stolichnaya . . . well, that works too.

Beyond ancient memories there are plenty of present-day thoughts that also deserve suppression. These range across the gamut of experience. You can think of a hundred for yourself if you pause from pushing them down. There are those which particularly trouble the physician, like the bad one of wondering when the lawyer for that patient-who-is-mad-at-you-for-absolutely-no-reason-whatsoever is going to be in touch, requesting all the records; or homely ones like the awareness that the shingles on the roof have gotten tired and worn and someone (like even the light-of-your-life wife) thinks they should be replaced pretty soon; or even quasi-good ones like the knowledge that your "child," who has maybe just gotten her driver's license, is even now for the first time driving herself and a whole gaggle of her friends down to the beach! Will one of the boys bring along beer or worse? No! You don't want to think about these things. And how about cleaning out the garage? One can simply go on and on about what one does not want to think about.

Not thinking takes, like any skill, a little practice, but one can become very proficient. Scarlett O'Hara may have had lots of neuroses but she could "not think" to a fine T. "No, I won't think about that," she said, "at least not today. I'll think about it tomorrow." Well said, I say.

That is exactly what I am doing myself. I am having a little operation. My delightful orthopedic surgeon, Dr. Donald Dewey, is going to axe off the heads of my grungy femurs. He is going to do some grinding about here and there, and after making the usual bloody orthopedic mess (ha! don't I sound like a real plastic surgeon?) plans to provide me with lovely, new Teflon and heavy metal joints. I asked him for guarantees, which he willingly gave me, that after the surgery my wife will adore me all the more. At least I will not, I hope, look like a crab in slow motion when I chase her, nor will she hear those grinding sounds, like gears failing to mesh, when I approach. I will become once again my former quick, young self, darting in to grab her, smooth and slick and quiet as a cat does a mouse.

My only fear, which of course I didn't think about, is the 1% incidence of infection. If this occurs I think you end up without a joint at all and have to kind of crawl about. Well, I've done a bit of that (thankfully suppressed in memory) in my time too, and could probably pick up that mode again fairly quickly.

But I simply made myself not think about that.

Nor will I think about the fact that if infection occurs such rare exotica as plastic surgeons might even be called in to consult. It seems to me, in such instances, that these dilettanti are then handed the opportunity, almost as on a silver salver, to invent or practice some huge, deforming flap that has to be lifted, slung about, and brought from some distant place to fill in the great black hole that is left once the poor hip bone is reamed out.

No, the idea of such an eventuality is not worth thinking about; I will shove that one right down into the old Red Nucleus[1] where, if my neuroanatomy serves, the worst of the unmemorable is stuffed.

In any case, none of this will happen. This is, after all, an almost perfect operation and Dr. D. is a veritable paragon of the compleat surgeon, debonair, etc., and knowing even his right hand from his left. It is almost worth having gravel, arrowheads, and probably even silicone lumps in my joints just to get to see his shining face in the morning when he comes to visit me on rounds.

It will be, as I tell my patients regarding their surgeries, "an adventure," and afterwards I will be able to cut my toenails again and put on my socks without standing on my head. I'm not going to think about the fact that Dr. D. says that I might, despite the surgery, not be able to put on my socks. I am going to think I will but, just in case I can't, I invented an ingenious device for putting socks on. I cleverly made it out of a wire clothes hanger, some clothespins, and a bit of string. I don't know why anyone wouldn't be delighted to use it. I'm going to call it the "Li'l Miracle Socker," advertise it on TV next to "Li'l Miracle Spot Remover," patent it, and become rich and famous.

So there, I do not need to think about anything else.

---

[1] A funny place in the brain where rage and other nonsense reside, I think!

Now I'm going to have lunch. It's Saturday so I see nothing wrong with asking my wife to join me for a bit of champagne, caviar and a crust, perhaps *al fresco* on the verandah.

But, drat, what is really just a porch is covered with wet and rotting leaves, which yesterday I decided I would not think about.

That's the worst thing about reality, sometimes it catches up with you, doesn't it?

PHLEBOTOMIZED
AND OTHER PLEASURES

*H*ave you done it all? Are you jaded by world-famous spas and casinos? Have you been everywhere, taken every tour, seen everything? Do you feel filled with an insufferable *fin de siècle ennui*? Does your heart yearn for a new kind of adventure, to fill its insatiable longing, and grant peace to your restless spirit?

Finally, do you think of yourself as being half an inch too short? Have you ever thought that life would be perfected if you saw it from the prospect of half an inch taller?

Well, for you and those of my friends similarly afflicted, I am recommending having both hips lopped off and replaced with heavy metal and some kind of Teflon derivative. If you have insurance it may well be cheaper than a vacation and far more exhilarating. All you have to do is pick a reasonably decent, or indecent, orthopedic surgeon . . . in my case none better than the estimable Dr. D. Dewey . . . who has in his drawer a standard set of x-rays of hip joints, demonstrating osteophytosis, aseptic necrosis, cystic horromata, and what look like Indian arrowheads and some trilobites.

In no time at all you're lying there watching some of your best friends give you Pentothol.

But the real fun, the adventure that really makes it worthwhile, starts after you wake up. My first recollection, back in my room, was of an enormous foam rubber pad between my legs. I have since (though adjured to use this device) found that our house cat does a great deal better job. As an abduction splint, once a cat snuggles down between your legs, there is simply no motion allowed. Wasn't it Mohammed who said, "Better to cut off the hem of thy garment than disturb a sleeping cat." Not bad theology.

As with most adventures, one starts off with fluffy ideas about just how everything is going to transpire, but inevitably the event proves altogether different from what you imagined. For one thing, total hip replacements have nothing to do with what "they" let out that "they" do. It is actually a matter of the surgeon simply pouring lead into your thighs while at the same time the anesthesiologist pumps everything out of your torso and brain-pan, replacing those contents with helium. You wake up wanting to float off, but your legs are like anchors, never mind the foam rubber shackles and the cat.

This perspective changes interestingly when you first try to get up, in my case on the second postoperative day. Although your thighs remain leaden, your head is bobbing up somewhere against the ceiling. You have the distinct impression that your acetabulae have been replaced with two thimbles and your femoral heads very delicately constructed of a glued pylon of toothpicks which articulate precariously into these thimbles. You are supposed to stand on this contraption and do because, after all, it's part of the adventure.

But it is not the surgery itself that so much defines the "adventure" as its peripheral spin-offs. Foremost amongst these is the delightful effect of an excellent phlebotomy. A hemoglobin of 6.5 may be just fine for lots of people, but for me it was heady stuff. It led me to rethink my position on those misguided centuries of phlebotomization when Byron and George Washington and everyone else were bled almost to death by their physicians, who quite unfairly now seem to us almost "quacks." In fact, a clean, quick loss of two or three pints of blood has about it something thoroughly exhilarating. It takes your mind off your condition. You are suddenly granted a lovely, lassitudinous perspective on the world and yourself. There is a slightly "out of body" feeling about it that I cannot but recommend highly. Then, of course, you gradually get to build back your hemoglobin level. As you do so you have the most delightful feeling of strength gathering, of improving, of getting somewhere, of being full of fresh, wholesome, brand-new, shiny blood. Scorn no longer, I say, the phlebotomists of yore.

Of course, there are some inconveniences; I mean the wretched creases in the bed, the muscle aches, inability to move, the headache, asthenia, curious sweats, strange fevers, the heel that simply will not get comfortable, the knee that aches, and eyes that burn. Inconveniences, peripheral and unimagined before the fact, very much enhance one's admiration for the courage of the chronically ill and infirm. But "it's not," as the wit said and was forever after repeated exasperatingly by one of my lesser uncles, "the cough that carries you off, it's the coffin they carry you offin'."

But surely my most dramatic moment was the day I first showered, three days postoperative. With the assistance of my excellent nurse, I managed to clamber into the tub and get seated on my little stool. Before turning the water on, as I sat there in a demi-dazed state, I felt a dreary feeling, vaporous and free floating. I knew that what blood I had was rushing even then to my toenails. "I think I'm going to faint," I said weakly, yet withal with a wee chuckle, just barely audible.

"Oh no," she exhorted me, "take deep breaths through your nose and let them out through your mouth!"

"What difference will that make?!" I barely managed to reply, because it was clear to me that my nose and everything else about me were rapidly vanishing.

I turned wonderfully pale, let me even say white as *blanc mange*, and forthwith fainted. But wait, it was better than mere syncope! I had drunk a whole can of V-8 juice 15 minutes before the episode and this, with colorful and dramatic effect, a veritable perfection of sudden internal hemorrhage, now emerged violently from my nose and mouth. It was a far better scene than the "Death of Marat" by Jacques Louis David. Marat simply lies dead in his tub, rather yellowish, without the brilliant colors of exsanguination.

I could not suppress a laugh when I woke. Poor Nurse Diana, on the other hand, had of course pulled all the emergency strings in the bathroom because she could scarcely guess what might come up next, but perhaps my liver, after the can of V-8 juice. But she survived it; as a matter of fact, she survived it rather well because she had herself given me the red draught and was able to make an accurate diagnosis of my colorful discharge. My recommendation, therefore, is that when you have this operation and drink a can of V-8 juice before you shower, don't tell the nurse.

In any case, I am on my way to recovery and can now take a shower all by myself without fainting. Pole vaulting anyone! Maybe next week!

What's left to say? Foremost is how extraordinarily kind and good people have been. Indeed, more than any vacation I have ever taken, this experience has been one of interest and enrichment. I have enjoyed the unprecedented opportunity to be quietly at home for two weeks. We have had some little "picnics." I have listened to music and played a little on the piano. My eye casts about our house and sees things of interest and beauty. I am reading aloud a Trollope novel to my wife as she sits and does some cross stitch. The cat sits between my legs purring. I am deeply grateful for the awareness that I am on the way to being fully restored and, as an immediate corollary, keenly sensitive to those who must in sickness endure so much worse, and with little hope in the outcome.

These awarenesses ain't bad.

And, by the way, I think I really am half an inch taller.

So bravo, Dr. Dewey, bravo the nurses, and bravo you all!

A CHART UNCHAINED

No, no, believe me! I am not one to suggest even remotely that the veritable Chart of any patient should be dealt with in even the least cavalier fashion. No, no, it should be treated with a salubrious seriosity, as befits the professional ethics of the medical practitioner and our high goal of bringing health to all mankind. As a further aside, we must also make sure that the chart is perfectly legible, ordered, tidy, and objectively factual so we may facilitate the work of the legal profession.

But there is always a "but." Granted, it is a little "but." But even so I want to say that in this huge world of impersonal computer jargon, of scientific facts that forbid even an occasional ingratiating adjective, and of legal tomes that reduce truth and passion to dry and crusty precedents, perhaps medicine just might . . . as the greatest of the humanitarian arts . . . be permitted an occasional modicum of humanity in our descriptions of disease and the human condition.

Well, operative reports and so on I grant must be exclusively factual, without flights of fancy or confabulation. But maybe, without denigration to the patient, it might be allowed from time to time that the practitioner of medicine interject into his notes something of the reality of the whole person, rather than just the condition or objective "problem."

I am led to think these revolutionary ideas as a result of having reviewed, as a member of the hospital's Utilization Review Committee, a chart the other day at one of those early morning breakfast meetings where we all love to review charts, while desperately hoping we can avoid eating a doughnut. In this case (would you believe it!) in the stack of charts before me I discovered . . . my own! My very own chart from eight weeks prior when I had both my hips replaced.

"Wow," thought I, "what a windfall. I will now see what that debonair and devilish orthopod of mine really thought about my progress."

Never minding the dull operative report, and the weighty masses of papers filled with remarks of not much meaning except for the solipsistic sake of the chart itself, I turned directly to my single and last outpatient visit with my surgeon to see what notes he made.

I cannot remember what I read, but like to imagine it was something as follows: "The patient returns as per his scheduled appointment, having missed five previously scheduled ones causing great inconvenience to ourselves."

"The patient is now seven weeks post-bilateral-hip-replacement. He is gimping around pretty well, brandishing a cane with a wicked looking bird-head handle. His gait without the cane is best described as 'lurching.' It is also 'lurching' with the cane. Patient describes his gait prior to the surgery as being 'lurching,' or more distinctly that of a 'drunken sailor.' He is content with this, having at one time been something of a drunken sailor, having grown fond of this mode of ambulation, which he thinks sets him off from the common herd of pigeon-toed walkers."

"I questioned him when he thought he might cease utilization of the cane. He replied that he has grown attached to it, because he has discovered that as an intermediary between himself and the calf of an attractive lady it works remarkably well. He notes that, as with ladies who find no offense in being patted on the tummy when they are pregnant, he can gently touch a pleasant calf with his cane . . . not to overdo it, and with discretion of course . . . and the maneuver is regarded with far more toleration than if he had used his hand. 'I think I'll stick with the stick,' he said. The patient is pleased with this aspect of his progress."

"He states he is bilaterally one-fourth to one-half an inch taller, which gives him a great deal more confidence, but is not so much that he has had to lengthen the hem on his trousers. He states that the incisions have done beautifully, and that these have in fact excited the admiration of his wife, who fondly calls them his 'racing stripes'. The scars are without any evidence of hypertrophy, and, if I may say so myself, are possibly the most beautifully healed scars I have ever seen. I have to agree with his wife myself, manly man that I am, that they are quite 'cute'."

"He states, with a somewhat libidinous leer, that he can now 'sneak up' (!) on his wife far better than heretofore, when he was given away by the grinding, clanking, and grating sounds that his hip joints made, and which always alerted her to his increasing proximity. He seems to think that there is some relationship between the titanium we have inserted and potency. Of course, he is a rather strange duck, and I would not be surprised if he does not present himself in due course asserting that during his surgery we not only replaced his hips but placed a radio receiver in his brain, and are dictating his behavior."

"X-ray examinations show the usual assortment of titanium, screws, nuts, bolts, cups, and, curiously, what looks like a broken saucer, but on one side only (need to check with my assistant Dr. what's-his-name, on what he put in there). On my side, as a passing note, there is a radiopaque strand suggesting a 4" x 4" sponge left in the depths of the wound. Given the quantity of artifact and hardware already *in situ*, this additional element should cause no problem."

"EXAM: Thighs flex, knees bend, and the gluteus muscles are present bilaterally. The scars are simply elegant."

"DISPOSITION: Continue to attempt chasing his wife, who can still just manage to escape him. He should be able to catch up to her in approximately two weeks. Use cane PRN, as needed, for whatever purpose. Make greater efforts towards more sober appearing gait pattern. Psychotherapy."

"Return in one week so I may feel his scars again and admire my work."

I sat back amazed, and ate a doughnut. "What a surgeon!" I thought. What a character, that he could write such fanciful things about little old me, and put it flat out in the chart, knowing that some Utilization Review Committee member might read it, or some JCAH[1] dignitary. And not give a twit! I read it through again, and fluffed my feathers with pride as I noted the incredible things he thought I might be capable of. He must be mad, but even so I was delighted. I passed the chart on forthwith, fully approved, with a note that his remarks had shown a nice concern for the whole man, fearlessly expressed if off the wall.

So home I went, pondering the curious impression I had made on a real, macho, orthopedic surgeon.

Goodness, it even crossed my mind to really try to "sneak up" on my wife!

---

[1]JCAH: The Joint Commission for Accreditation of Hospitals, a living remnant of the former Soviet NKVD.

BOUQUETS OF CLICHÉS[1]

T rue, at dinner the other night the very fact that we were trying to get our 10-year-old daughter to eat something green has to be considered a modern parental cliché. In Dickens' time nothing was green, and the cliché was that a dose of treacle at bedtime quite sufficed.

Even worse as a cliché, I added insult to injury by actually making a remark about "the poor African children who do not have enough to eat." My attempt was no more effective as when, in tried and true fashion, my own parents attempted to get me, at age 10, to eat something green by citing "the starving Chinese."

Thoroughly thwarted and my arguments unheard, I lapsed into quiet reverie, rolling my eyes across the table at my wife. (Not literally, of course, but kind of like a cliché itself.)

But I couldn't bear it. After all, we were all gathered together for dinner, the older daughter home from college on spring break, the two cats dozing about on the dining room floor, and the two dogs ever eager that some morsel might drop out of our mouths and into theirs. It was my job "made stale by usage" (Webster's definition of a "cliché") to make sure we had a lively, intelligent, mind-expanding, and informative conversation. What's a Dad for at the dinner table otherwise?

---

[1] *cliché:* Fr., p.p. of cliché, variant of *cliquer* to click applied by die sinkers to the striking of melted lead to obtain a proof or cast. Hence the name applied to a stereotype block or "dabs."

I tried "What is the best thing that happened to you today?" and "What is the worst . . . ?" but everyone was very loathe to commit themselves, and in any case scarcely knew. Once more, into the breech, I tried to get things rolling by answering the question myself, but found I scarcely knew either. The best I could conjure for the "best thing" that had happened was that a patient had brought us three dozen country eggs, unfertilized and capable of hatching into little chickens, delivered into my arms with a grateful speech. The worst thing that had happened was that we discovered that we have a rather longer way to go than I had thought to get our quarterly tax payment together by April 15th. When you get right down to it, none of that was very interesting, although I tried to throw in lots of curlicues, footnotes, asterisks, and clever asides, mostly more clichés, to make it so.

My wife and I, to demonstrate that conversation is possible between consenting adults, chatted at her instigation about the dogwood coming into bloom: How lovely to see those fine points of white just coming out, clear and dainty, all over town and in the deep woods. Suddenly a tree that you never see otherwise, that fades totally into the background, and that you scarcely recognize when not in bloom, cries forth, making an exclamatory statement that, no matter how repetitive, each spring never seems a cliché.

"Aha," thought I, warming to the subject, and presenting aloud my sudden perception, "we are all of us just like dogwoods. Against the great backdrop of nature, time, and events, we are scarcely visible, seem to make no difference much whatsoever, and yet every now and then, maybe, most of us burst into bloom over something!" I became eloquent, or what I think is eloquent, but which usually ends up being something that might border more on the incomprehensible. But no matter; a man's home is his castle, as the cliché tells us, and in his own dining room, within the loving bosom of his family and surrounded by his own cats and dogs, one can get away with a lot so long as you don't fidget too much, or throw your food.

Accordingly I carried on. Indeed, I carried on in fine fettle: "We are all poised and pregnant with the capacity for a grand blossoming but are thwarted by the huge effort it takes, after all, to bloom. Certainly 'April is the cruelest month'; it is much easier to amble on in the usual fashion, treading the same well-trodden path, seeing only what we have always seen, swept on by the tide of events, and stopping not to smell the roses. Our lives . . . ," waving my spoon in the hopes that I would attract the attention of the teenager and preteen, "are nothing more than our own choice of clichés, strung together in such fashion as to define our personalities as uniquely as our dermatoglyphics, almost as characteristic a sequence as that of amino acids in the structure of DNA. Little enough do we play a wild card, or come up with a mutant remark that incorporates within itself the bright light of revelation. Oh, mundane are our lives, and mundanely we tread the well-known paths . . . etc."

No one can bear much of this. The 10-year-old actually ate her two green beans and, in desperation, asked if she might be excused from the table. The teenager suddenly had to telephone a friend. My wife and I sipped our wine, surrounded by the cats and dogs who remained faithful through all. Yet the banal has a life of its own, and so we steadfastly did the dishes, and shared a hug. We are used to our family patterns.

I am used to my professional ones as well, even, I suppose, to guarding them rather jealously. It is my preference to be left alone in my practice, nestled down in my delightful little office with a fridge full of junk food, doing what I can for folks here and there, making a pleasant living, and being content with the eggs I have been given. Every now and then I get to do something slightly out of the ordinary, or even almost have a flash of insight, or a thought that is more a bloom than a cliché. I had one a couple of weeks ago, I really did, but not having written it down I forgot it, and that bright blossom is gone forever. I wonder what it was.

Yet if I am content behind the bastion of my own clichés, both personal and professional, I fear that the latter are retreating before the vastly more powerful onslaught of other clichés, namely those of the HMOs, coming at us like bullets. Our cherished images of the independent old doctor, like Doc in "Gunsmoke," are becoming as anachronistic as the clichés of shoot-outs on the streets of Dodge. The clichés we speak in defense of how medicine has been practiced in the past are crouched tensely at the line of scrimmage opposite the clichés of a new and now politically powerful version of health-care delivery. We cry "patients first," "the best in the world," "the greatest advances," and "down with the lawyers;" their cheerleaders chant "access for all," "down with the costs," "guaranteed insurability," and "managed competition."

Who knows what will be achieved out of all this; but come what may, I am going to struggle to believe that "everything will be all right," because, after all, as the French put it, "*le plus ça change, le plus tout reste la même chose*." I take comfort in this happy homily that change is more perception than reality because, if the French say it, especially in French, doesn't it have to be true?

And don't forget that business about "nothing to fear but fear itself," and how about "when there is life, there is hope."

I will cling, like the drowning man grasping at a straw, to my own set of comforting clichés. I will even take comfort in the little known cliché that says (if not in French) that no matter what they do to us, we physicians will still be the blossoms on the health-care tree.

And spring always follows winter.

And it's always darkest before the dawn.

Etc., choose your own, in any language.

⎡ A C L S [1] Y E S ⎤

⚘

Every now and then . . . not every two years as recommended, but maybe every three . . . I seem to gather my resources together to learn, once again, more or less, where the heart is.

I do this by getting recertified in ACLS. It requires giving up a whole invariably glorious and balmy weekend, but once done my doubts are cast aside. Once again I can bask in the illusion that I know something about how the heart ticks and tocks, and which comes first, and what drugs to give if it tick-tick-ticks rather than tick-tocks, or whether under what circumstances to just give it a big kick with a few hundred jewels (ha! I really know it's Joules) lying handily around. This is all very good for me and good discipline too, which my children tell me I need. But I do not kid myself into thinking I know anything much about how to resuscitate anybody beyond just barely myself in the morning when I get out of bed. In my office, thank-God-and-let-us-not-even-mention-the-fact, I have never had any horror that my primary resuscitative technique, namely the Trendelenburg position,[2] didn't pretty quickly correct.

---

[1]Advanced Cardiac Life Support, or how to start your heart when it stops by using the utmost latest applications, algorithms, and drugs.

[2]An unnatural "head-down, tail-up" position contrary to that of the healthy tadpole (see "Requiem for a Cookie," in the "Homely" section of this book) tried and true for bringing people back from a faint by almost instantly draining from your legs, elevated now higher than your heart, two units of blood to your poor brain. This causes you to wake up and feel better quick.

As a matter of fact, my success with this old maneuver makes me wonder why the Trendelenburg inversion isn't much more highly touted in ACLS and BLS[3] than it is. It has invariably worked for me. Sad to say we are getting away from the good old "precordial thump," which always seemed appealing in its brute simplicity (but is now thought to be quite "optional"), but on the other hand this maneuver simply does not compare to turning someone upside down and giving them a good shake, thus flushing out all the blood in their legs and making it go to their brain and activating all those reticular centers and basilar elements that set everything right again. I like the part, too, when the patient afterwards asks, "Why am I upside down?" and you reply "Oh well, a little technical problem with the table that we'll set right quick as a bunny." Then you straighten them out and carry on with whatever you are doing, remarking blithely about what a beautiful day it is.

Yes, this has always worked like a charm for me, but ACLS accreditation seems (as Captain Hook used to say, starring Dustin Hoffman and Robin Williams) "Good form."

So I got accredited once again, and have survived, and have my little ACLS Accomplishment button, which I will probably lose tomorrow.

Even if I lose it, I was delighted to get it, although I had some fears on the point. Much has changed in just the last three years in terms of guidelines for advanced resuscitation. I was afraid they might have discontinued giving us the button, not only for cost containment reasons but more importantly because in some terrible legal way the possession of a button might put the American Heart Association in jeopardy, as if they had given us the right to go around resuscitating people and giving them electric shocks. Then, if the patient died despite all you had done, including putting them upside down, the AHA could be named in the suit. But no, gratify-

---

[3]Basic Life Support, or how to start your heart when it stops by using more casual methods than ACLS.

ingly, you still get a button, although you do sign lots and lots of stuff that says this does not mean you think yourself, or anyone else thinks you, expert or even qualified, in all the little techniques they teach you. God knows, I certainly would not be so rash as to think it!

In any case, at least I know where the heart is again and can, with 50% accuracy, using a kind of eeny-meenie-miney-mo technique, tell a Mobitz I[4] from a Mobitz II.[5] I also learned in the course that there is some stuff called "Easy Red," which soaks up all manner of liquid and turns it instantly into a blob. It is highly touted for all the things we deal in such as blood, urine, and vomit, as well as being good for cleaning up after domestic animals, dogs, cats, horses, and maybe even cows. Someone put some in my coffee and turned it instantly into a disgusting coagulum, which you could hardly look at without getting arrhythmic.

On the last morning, our long-suffering and stoical instructors tested us individually. Most of the things you have to do to pass come fairly second nature to any physician of a slightly thoughtful bent. Nonetheless it is a little nervous trying to remember all those algorithms. Everyone else is watching you with narrowed pupils as you desperately scratch around in the hope that you will hit upon the right formula and regurgitate a proper curd. The teaching method this time around seemed more helpful in avoiding this debacle, and the whole process of resuscitation actually made some kind of sense.

Of further interest with respect to the course were the demonstrations of a new defibrillator. It happily almost leaves you the option of not having to have any "sense" at all, nor do you even have to sort a mess of cables and paddles and hope that they're all set up. You simply put on a little sticky pad and the rest is history. The computer voice from the defibrillator soothingly tells you to "wake up," "look at the patient," "take courage," or do what seems necessary from the computer's point of view. But still, just like pilots

[4]A squiggle on an electrocardiogram.
[5]Another squiggle or something.

in their computerized aircraft, we physicians like to have ultimate control, so happily the semiautomatic computer arranges for you to push a button when it says "push." This is very wonderful, the only catch being that while the computer is talking to you it is also recording everything you say so that it can send a tape immediately to the patient's lawyer when you are finished. Accordingly you have to be very careful not to say all those "bleep" things that Richard Nixon used to say on his tapes, and for goodness sake sound like you are in some vague command of yourself. I deepened my voice as best I could, trying to sound like a doctor on a soap opera. I think this worked pretty well and surely helped me pass the exam.

Last, but not to be stuffy or proudful, it was interesting to me that amongst the great gaggle of people taking this course most were nurses, EMT technicians, and otherwise. Out of about 50 people there were only four physicians. Well, I suppose cardiologists know all this stuff, and emergency room doctors, and maybe just barely even anesthesiologists and dermatologists. But it is an illumination to us plastic surgeons.

In any case, for the moment I think I almost know something about kicking the heart into action and hope to retain it for at least 48 hours. Meanwhile, to boot, I'm going to keep my eye out closely for a Mobitz I or II, make the diagnosis in a rich baritone if one comes my way, and immediately put the patient into Trendelenburg position.

If that doesn't work, I hope I don't faint.

CLINICAL DIAGNOSIS, BRILLIANT AND NOT SO

When I was growing up the only flavor of physician I knew or had any contact with was our GP. We had two doctors in our little town. One was young and just barely back from World War II, and the other was old by my estimates at the time, respected if not venerable, and lived in a great big white house with awnings. He had something of an old family name in the county. Of course, he was our doctor.

I had very little, if any, conception that medicine might be composed of "specialists." But by report there was an exotic species of physician 170 miles north in St. Louis whom everyone called a "diagnostician," as in "He is a Diagnostician." Actually the description of this sublunar person was almost invariably rendered in the superlative: "He is a brilliant diagnostician." I pictured this character with difficulty, sometimes seeing him as an ordinary mortal but on other occasions dressed in veritable cloth of gold. In my imagining he was a person perfectly in command of himself, imperturbable, and going about doing nothing but laying his eyes and hands on the bafflingly ill, to come up with a "brilliant" and always correct diagnosis of some strange disease that confounded everyone else. He would accept the plaudits of ordinary GPs with graceful detachment before moving on to shower his expertise elsewhere. Never did he deign to treat a single person, such an exercise being scarcely worth his intellect.

I doubt, although I am still not absolutely sure so strong are childhood impressions, that such a beast as a "Diagnostician" ever existed. But in the landscape of my memory this glittering bird left, contrary to reason, a residuum of fine feathers; namely, that I could never be one. Oh, granted, I have never been so thoroughly lacking in diagnostic skills that I ever started intravenous fluids on a lifeless body, as the odd intern is famous for having done; but probably I was just lucky. But if I have lucked out in never having misdiagnosed "Death," I have always rather dreaded situations requiring too great an assortment of differential diagnoses.

In medical school I enjoyed the rudiments of "Clinical Diagnosis" but thereafter loathed and despised those awkward moments, on rounds grand or otherwise, when you were supposed to glibly come up with a long list of Esoterica that must be ruled out hither and thither, and in my nervousness usually left out or overlooked most of the obvious and almost all of the esoteric. Utilizing the usual forms of BS, ending on a light and merry note, I thought I got away with it all pretty well. Maybe I did. I passed in any case. But that doesn't mean I liked it much.

As a matter of fact, one of the reasons, the unromantic reason, that I went into plastic surgery was because there did not seem to be a lot of diagnosis involved. No, as I saw it the skin sits there in all its glory, regulating with marvelous if little acknowledged insouciance the internal *milieu* (or the *milieu intèrieur* since the French described it) and protecting one from the horrors of the outside world. For all practical purposes, never minding abstruse forms of dermatopathology, there is no more to diagnose than a wrinkle, a bump, or a hole. On these I can pounce and, to some modest degree, even "fix." I don't even have to go through those elaborate exercises that so appeal to the dermatologist: Although I can spell "pityriasis," I do not bandy the term around loosely nor any of their other arcane diagnoses, rendered in what I consider the last bastion of the Latin language in medical usage.

Secretly, of course, I harbor an admiration for the "brilliant" clinical diagnostician, most particularly that member of "the older school" who, with stethoscope and palpating finger, can come up with an answer even before the trolley comes to fetch the poor patient to the CT scanner.

Along such diagnostic lines I can only remember having had one victorious experience, which is related only as an introduction to my most recent diagnostic debacle. This experience is very briefly put: It occurred in the emergency room when I was called in to look at the victim of an automobile accident and sew up some lacerations on her face. I thought she looked awfully pale given the relatively minor extent of the lacerations, and when she said she had a pain in her left shoulder when she breathed I pounced on it more or less, and discovered that her left upper quadrant was a little tight and tender. Restraining my enthusiasm, I reported my suspicions of splenic rupture to the emergency room physician. He came into the room and after a mere glance and quick feel rewarded me with a kind of pleasant grunt. It was all in a day's work to him, but I thought I had quite probably saved a life. I also plugged up a hole in the poor skin.

On the other hand I have just recently had an experience rather less than "brilliant" as a "diagnostician." Having puffed myself up over diagnosing the ruptured spleen, I am now cast down and am humble. The experience demonstrates clearly that everywhere lie pitfalls in clinical diagnosis, primrose paths down which I for one am delighted to skip without the least second glance at the glaring facts.

The diagnostic challenge occurred as I drove our two daughters back from Charlotte, North Carolina, where they had been visiting family. The older, age 19, who has long ago learned the skills of putting on makeup in a moving vehicle, was doing just that when she confronted me with the following:

"Daddy (how pleasant that she still calls me that), one of my eyes is bigger than the other!" To this sort of observation I am inured. I hear it all the time about people's nostrils, or their ear lobes, or for heaven's sake indeed even their breasts, and am quite readily prepared with an answer to the effect that clearly our maker never guaranteed that our contralateral halves would be exactly the same.

"Oh well," I said, "you probably just got one of your eyes from your Mom and the other from me."

"No, I don't mean the eye, I mean the little black hole in the eye."

"Oh, you mean the pupil," I replied, glancing askance at her.

She turned to look at me quite hard,[1] her eyelids wide open. It took a mere askance glance to notice that her pupil on the right was widely dilated and the one on the left rather small.

"Good heavens!" I cried, "put your eyeball down there in the light and let me see what happens."

She did so, and there was not a flicker of motion in the pupil. My daughter had a "fixed, dilated pupil," and I remembered from clinical diagnosis that this was bad.

Never mind the lack of headache or any other signs or symptoms. My daughter clearly had some terrible brain tumor, something I probably had forgotten even how to spell, and it had wound its way around her oculomotor system and had probably already invaded the Limbics, not to mention that wretched Red Nucleus. Of course I remained quite calm, but knocked up the cruise control a couple of miles per hour, the better to get home to my friend the ophthalmological surgeon and brilliant diagnostician.

"Hello, Tony," I said, after getting him on the phone. "My daughter has a fixed dilated pupil, which we just noted on our drive back from Charlotte."

There was only a moment's pause.

"Does she have on a scopolamine patch? Look behind her right ear." I didn't need to look. I had given her one a few days before for this very trip.[2]

---

[1] If you made the correct diagnosis in the paragraph beginning "She turned to look at me quite hard," you are a "Brilliant Diagnostician" like Dr. Tony Weaver. If you did not make the diagnosis, you should apply to a plastic surgery residency and learn to diagnose more obvious things like cleft lip.

[2] Scopolamine is helpful in combatting motion sickness. It also, like atropine, and "belladonna" (beautiful lady indeed!) dilates the pupil. Even if I had remembered the patch I did not dream the effect on the pupil would be so profound.

But I had forgotten. They had never taught me to think of that in my clinical diagnosis course.

As for myself and our old family GP, I take it as a lesson that he had merely given me enemas for my ruptured appendix for three days until I went into a coma and became anuric. We got the new doctor, who had no awnings on his house, but who diagnosed a board-like abdomen and rushed me off to a "brilliant country surgeon."

I thoroughly lived, and my daughter's pupil went down to normal after a couple of days.

But give me a hole in the skin any day.

ROMANCING THE STONE

I t has recently come to my attention that the world is not made of *Earth, Air, Fire, and Water. It is made of only two primordial elements: Glitz and Stones.*

I have been in receipt of this information as a result of recent communication with Sam Rosenthal, MD, who, despite being possessed of a sufficient personal style, quite disparages glitz, particularly when spelled with a capital G. Forgive me, given the time and space constraints imposed upon this essay, that I do not elaborate upon the essential differences between small g "glitz" and Glitz. Let my meaning suffice that if Dr. Rosenthal has a distinctive enough manner he is also a hard-rock, down-to-earth thinker, more interested in the long-term Verities, Platonic Forms, getting the basics right, and all that. He is the kind of man, and with sufficient displacement too, so that if he, like Samuel Johnson, were to kick a stone he might with equal power intone (he has a Johnsonian voice), "thus I refute Berkeley," or in this case glitziness. I am paraphrasing him because I did not take notes during our meeting, but I think he said (there was no stone around to kick), "It's real things that matter, not this *%*#*! X#*&+⁰!@#$ Glitz!" (I don't know if he really said "*$&*@" either).

Even if he can kick a stone better than I, who lack all that mass and am limited by substitute titanium hips, I was nonetheless quick to agree, noting that there was enough Glitz in the world already without physicians adding to it further.

Of course, some of you might wonder how two plastic surgeons (indeed!) can take such a position on Glitz. After all, we are supposed to

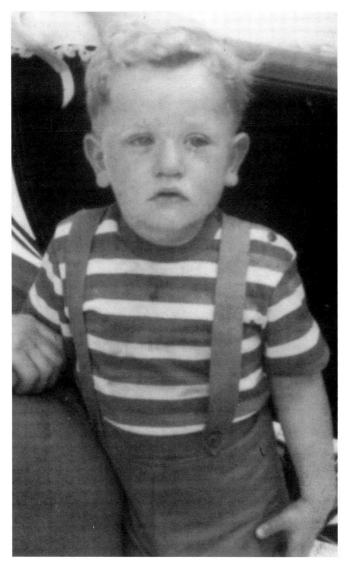

Dr. Rosenthal as an unbelievably unglitzy, small, and slightly out of focus child.

be fairly full of frivolity, and practice a glitzy kind of half surgery so "unnecessary" that insurance doesn't even cover it much of the time. I remember about 20 years ago reading an article in *Time* magazine on a plastic surgery meeting in Hollywood, Florida. In the most deprecatory terms, the writer made merry with descriptions of beautifully coifed plastic sur-geons mincing about in their "bell bottoms" and other glitz. Well, I wasn't at that meeting and never wore bell bottoms because they made me look too short. But the article hurt my feelings. Anyway I have always taken a bit of umbrage about this image of plastic surgeons, although I guess there are those who live up to it, but surely only in places far away and long ago like New York and California.

In any case, I was inspecting Dr. Rosenthal's office and surgery for qual-ity assurance and accreditation purposes, and immediately found myself comforted by the wholesome matter-of-fact state of his premises. All was as Q.A. would have it, although for completeness' sake I noted certain things on the posting of the escape routes from his office in case of fire. Having been cited for delinquencies on this item myself, I have now become fierce on the point. Because his office, like mine, is small and on the ground floor with lots of windows and doors, I suggested a comprehensive map with red arrows boldly going out every window and door. I realize, on the other hand, that there are some offices (and this is not to impugn them as glitzy) located on the 15th floor of high-rise buildings, which need perforce a more comprehensive approach. But I have never inspected one of these and so cannot be authoritative or adviceful.

In any case, we went through the handbook for accreditation and ticked off all the many, many pages of items that are supposed to be oper-ating and on site, not leaving out the fact that the baseboards in the oper-ating room must be four inches high and "roll up." I did not think it was glitzy of Dr. Rosenthal, by the way, when he rather proudly showed me his fulfillment of this requirement. When I next do an inspection, I will take along a ruler, however.

Finished with the exam, I wished to prolong the pleasure of my stay in the midst of such cheery, good company as himself and his delightful staff. Accordingly, as I looked at the books in his office, I thought I would ask

Dr. Rosenthal which one had been to him the most important in his medical career. It proved to be a standard, stony work, and led into his reciprocal query about which book was the most seminal influence in my career choice.

I have a ready response to this question. When I was a second-year medical student I stumbled on Dr. Ralph Millard's rare and idiosyncratic biography-history-surgical text relating to Sir Harold Gillies who, in meeting the challenge of devastating facial injuries in World War I, founded the plastic surgery specialty. This unique volume (I and II) decided me on plastic surgery as a career, the decision reinforced by my contact that same year with Hal Bingham, MD, now retired as Professor and Chief of Plastic Surgery at Shands Teaching Hospital and a recipient of the prestigious Pickrell Award for the excellence of his teaching. Some might think that reconstructing a shattered, machine-gunned face using tube pedicle flaps in 1916 was "Glitzy," but I considered it the veritable romancing of stern, stony, harsh reality. As for Dr. Bingham, no one who knows him has ever accused him of glitz, even with a little g, and even though he plays a mean jazz clarinet.

In my last essay I wrote in passing about the "nonromantic" reasons I went into plastic surgery, namely, because I was intimidated by "Clinical Diagnosis." By the time I left Dr. Rosenthal's office, I thought it would be only fair to note the more compelling reason I went into it: the machine-gunned faces of those young men and the ideal of their rehabilitation through reconstructive surgery.

Never mind that it has not quite worked out as my romantic idealism then dreamed, and that I find myself doing routine plastic surgical things, including very nonglitzy warts, in a fairly humble setting, while meanwhile trying not to snack too much between times. The hard face of reality always intervenes, but behind that reality the romance of the images that led me (I want to say all of us) into our various fields, into medicine itself, lingers on and gives strength, at least to me. So I think does Withering for the cardiologist; Hunter or Halstead, the surgeon; Morgagni, the pathologist; Osler, the internist; Madam Curie, the radiologist; Benjamin Rush, never minding his phlebotomizing, the psychiatrist; Sims, the gynecologist; and, of course, Nils Rosen von Rosenstein, the pediatrician. In hard and glitzy times these people are the stones that ballast us and keep the ship upright.

There is nothing of glitz in the romance of an ideal.

Nor in Dr. Rosenthal. As Inspector of his facility, I ticked off the hard objective facts—the oximeter, the defibrillator, etc.—finding all the stones in their place.

When I said good-bye and shook Dr. Rosenthal's hand, it was nonetheless pleasant not only to know how nicely his bits and pieces were in place but how pleasant had been the shared rapport between two physicians, still able to romance the old stones in spite of the bureaucrats, restraints, regulations, and penalties.

As for my own baseboards, God help me, they're only three and a half inches high, which I will keep secret.

YES, I AM
A DOCTOR

Plastic surgeons are thought to be notorious for their reclusive ways. Our Society, The American Society of Plastic and
Reconstructive Surgeons, not infrequently regales us on this topic,
deploring our building elaborate facilities, complete with intercom
systems and telephones in the bathrooms, yet withdrawing from the medical
community at large and, generally speaking, giving the impression of doing
curious, to some even suspect, deeds in our private operating "suites." Students
of our "image" find us to be even a bit standoffish and conceivably egocentric.

Real doctors, who regulate people's insulin dosages and take out colon
cancers, may not even have a very good idea of what it is we might do
beyond the fact that it probably isn't very necessary. The result is, just perhaps, that on the spectrum of medical care-giving, if surgeons and internists
are smack dab in the middle, with pediatricians and gastroenterologists on
either side, and folks like radiologists and pathologists to the left and right
of them, plastic surgeons are way off yonder to the right, barely much closer
to the center than perhaps chiropractors just over the horizon to the left.

All of the above, of course, is a gross generalization, and I myself have
never quite come to terms with it all. As for my relationships in the medical community, I prefer the lusty shouts of Aramis, Porthos, D'Artagnan,
and Athos: "All for one and one for all!"

This does not contradict that one can be permitted a touch of reclusive-
ness. Some of us truly are more apt to be startled by a loud noise, for example, made by some other more robust surgeon, and are verily content to

keep a low profile. Interestingly, I think I am at my best with urologists. In any case, whatever my "reclusive" inclinations, they seem to me fairly forgivable. After all, when I have been startled by the loud noise of the aforementioned surgeon, I do honestly take a certain delight in the clamor, and am pleased to see others manfully (excuse me ladies) oaring through the deep waters of life.

On the other hand, our society tells us we should moil and broil more with other physicians, be good fellows, and maybe even teach them by hook or crook that we, too, actually practice a form of medicine and surgery. I am not altogether sure how well I can succeed in moiling, and hope that those of my colleagues whom I (rarely) bump into in the hospital will forgive me if I suddenly make uncharacteristic remarks as I attempt to broil my way nearer the center of the medical spectrum, toward that point where I perceive they (hallelujah!) stand.

Actually, when you come right down to it, the only time I ever get to practice these endeavors are on those (occasional) occasions when I have a surgery in the hospital as opposed to in my elaborate suite under the old oak tree, surrounded by a picket fence, with only two telephone lines, a nasty computer, and mere three and a half inch baseboards.

At the hospital I have the great pleasure of seeing at least an aliquot of anesthesiologists. These ladies and gentlemen I always perceive as very lively, perhaps in counterpoint to the fact that they are usually making everyone else moribund in their professional endeavors. Like the urologists, they are full of gossip and merry. It is from them that I learn most of what I know about what may be going on in the hospital: What underhanded activity, what skullduggery, what treachery, what amazement, and so on. For someone like myself, rarely exposed to these revelations, it is all pretty heady stuff.

After my "case," however, the icing comes when I get to have a bowl of soup and a sandwich in the surgeons' lounge. There I find the best of the musketeers: General surgeons, orthopods, and pathologists slurping their soup and tossing lettuce leaves covered with Russian dressing at each other. I try pretty hard to "fit in" as I imagine one ought. The group is generally sufficiently heterogeneous that even the shyest plastic surgeon can usually find a chink into which to slip. I have a good time, for after all where could I find more delightful associations than with Dr. Woody Burgert, a great gentleman of, almost, "the old school" and wry of wit; Dr. Alberto Cola, who looks like Rudolph Valentino and has the added panache, which Valentino didn't, of coming from Uruguay; and Dr. Ralph Zimmerman, who has a curiously shrewd sort of thought process but camouflages it with an off-handed sense of irony. All of these people have wonderful things often enough to say, and even say them sometimes between spoonfuls of soup.

I am honored enough to work modestly at "fitting in" and even chirping up with some little *soupçon* that I just barely conceive as noteworthy, hoping to sound, as well, slightly rumbustious. Of course, I finish off by tossing a few lettuce leaves of my own, covered with goop, before retreating to my office.

But is it enough? Does it satisfy my Society?

I rather doubt it.

Therefore, for the sake of that group I am writing this so they will know up there in Chicago, where we plastic surgeons have our windy headquarters, that I am doing my best to fit in and be amalgamated. I simply can do no more. Aside from which, though I believe indeed we must all stick together, I don't think our Society needs be so paranoid about how we plastic surgeons may be perceived. After all, we are all of us struggling to achieve something happy for people, and if plastic surgeons don't deal quite so much in matters of life and death, we certainly do on occasion and, in any case, perhaps more than any specialty, consider closely the meaning of form, function, and (yes!) the "Quality of Life."

Therefore, if I only have the pleasure of the company of my numerous medical colleagues rarely, I send them my best regards and thank them too that I may take the pleasure, when in their company, of seeing myself as a really, truly

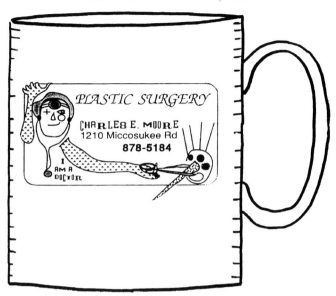

physician, speaking the language of one for all even if I don't know, offhand, the normal lab values for antiglomerular basement membrane antibodies.

So, on behalf of our Society, I beg that you consider us as "doctors," and if we are not as merry as urologists and anesthesiologists, it is only because we are burdened by the pressures that Art imposes, as well as being only one level below the neurosurgeon in terms of the cost of our liability premium.

Surely that alone qualifies one to say, "I am a doctor." And if that is not suffi-cient, I, at least, have a custom-created business card sent me by a (happy!) patient, a designer, who thought my lack of business cards a flaw . . . and so cre-ated for me a set, and had one blazoned, for all to see, on my own coffee cup.

"I am a doctor."

And I think it a privilege.

STRANGE, THE STRANGE ATTRACTOR

While on the subject of being a real doctor I suppose I quite qualify after all, because . . .

The fact is that about three or four months ago I was sewing up the thumb of some poor, unfortunate drunken soul in the middle of the night, and in so doing pierced my dermal integrity with the needle.

The patient, of course, was HIV positive and under treatment for fairly florid manifestations of AIDS. The result of this penetrating little episode was that I became immediately uncommonly thoughtful.

Now let me tell you that in the course of my modest surgical career, I have pointedly stabbed and sliced myself from time to time. Perhaps sometimes it has been a little bit my fault, but sometimes, as in this case, it pretty much wasn't. In any case, I was applying the strictest set of OSHA[1] regulations to my care of this gentleman, who all the personnel in the emergency room had quietly informed me possessed the deadly virus. The middle of the night, however, with an inebriated, rather hyperactive individual flailing about the emergency room, is not a particularly ideal place to be applying what, laughably I rather think, are called "universal precautions."

Well, I had discovered the ends of the severed extensor tendon to this person's thumb and had made a few passes here and there with my needle, attached of course to the suture material. As luck would have it, or the moon, or more certainly the Strange Attractor, the needle lay off to my left,

[1]OSHA: Occupational Safety and Health Administration.

among the drapes, having fallen in just such a way so that it was pointed straight up. Having tied a knot, I swept my left hand across the drapes and felt the distinct stabbing into the flesh.

Never mind that it is at least a little bit known that it takes a modest dose of HIV-infected blood to become infected. One wants even so to say a strong four-letter word, but I contented myself with a "damn!" (four letter indeed) under the breath, because I had a couple of premedical students assigned to the emergency room watching my every move under stress. Accordingly I made no disclosure of the fact that I had been stuck, not at 1:30 in the morning wanting to do any hand-wringing with them or create the necessity of expounding on universal precautions, OSHA regulations and the incidence of health-care providers becoming infected. All I wanted was to go home and have a glass of cold milk and a peanut butter and jelly sandwich, which is what I did.

On the way home, however, I remained altogether thoughtful.

How strange is that coincidence of events that can occur and which can be so vital in one's life depending upon the manner in which mind and matter will sometimes converge to so sharp a focus, so sharp indeed that matters even unto life and death may hang in the balance. I thought, as I drove, how extraordinary it was that all space and time in the universe should so conspire that here and there, now and again, we kind of meet our fate. What is, I thought to myself, the "Strange Attractor"? What is it that conspires, out of all eternity, to drive one man into a 7–11 and buy at just precisely the right moment just precisely the right ticket to win the lottery? And another to get stuck with a needle?

I thought of my own experience in medical school when a "great surgeon" (truly) decided, at the end of a very long case during which I supported a retractor, to biopsy the pancreas. Major things had already been achieved in the depths of the duodenum and the ampulla of Vater[1]; strictures had been

---

[1] Abraham Vater, 1684-1751, a German anatomist who described not only "Vater's fold," wherever that may be, but also that little pucker that marks the opening of the bile duct as it enters the duodenum.

dealt with, loops brought up, ostomies performed, and for all I can remember the vena cava shunted off some place. It had taken a long time and gone simply beautifully. The patient's circumstance looked very good indeed. Perhaps, however, I just thought it looked "good indeed" because I was exhausted and wild to get out of there, to fly to the Coke machine and its neighbor, that dispenser of those terrible orange crackers filled with pseudo–peanut butter for which you acquire an avid taste during medical school and residencies.

But the great surgeon said those fatal words, beads of sweat having been mopped from his brow: "Let's take a biopsy of the pancreas before we close."

Oh, let's indeed! Everything in the entire history of the universe since the Big Bang had conspired to bring that surgeon and that patient together at that point, in which we call this moment in time, and had further refined the point to suggest that the surgeon contemplate biopsying a very particular spot in the head of the pancreas. Another surgeon might not have contemplated the act, but this one did, distilling his decision out of the fluxes and flows of the seemingly random atoms in the universe that had gathered about him and this patient, and even little old me. How beautiful it was that we should all have been exactly where we were, and yet how unpredictable the next moment: Just like the marvel of an electron, which somehow or other contrives to be here and not here all at once, the reckoning of its reality in space changed almost by the very thought of it, in the twinkling of a nanosecond the biopsy needle was in the great surgeon's hands.

He, deep in the science of his profession, marvelously respected and honored and having committed long ago to memory the previous 50 years of every issue ever published of *Annals of Surgery* and the *New England Journal of Medicine*, performed the biopsy.

Blood hit the overhead light almost immediately and everyone almost fainted, at least I almost did. I was not used to such things, having been brought up in a nice home. Absolutely everything went to pieces, or in common parlance chaos reigned. A finger was quickly plunged toward the hole, which further gaped, and suddenly the entire abdominal cavity was simply full of blood. Let me not trouble you with morbid descriptions that none of us want to hear. Suffice it to say that the patient quite died.

As I drove home I thought of all this and the book I did after all finish, *Chaos* by James Glieck, which featured this marvelous entity, the "Strange Attractor." I suppose it is comforting to know that it is this that somehow or other results in so much that occurs to us. It is the Strange Attractor that through all time and history led the Titanic to hit that iceberg. It is this that causes you to decide before jumping in your car to go back into the house to get some trifle, that trifling pause resulting in your either having a horrible lethal accident or not having a horrible lethal accident. Within this concentration of space and time, the Strange Attractor, like the Phantom of the Opera, is there to lead the winner of the lottery to buy just the right ticket at just the right 7–11.

I suppose, as we practice medicine and life, we do actually hope, as through a glass, very, very darkly, to weave our way somehow or other between the various agglutinations of matter and energy that the Strange Attractor brings to focus, hoping in the midst of what seems chaos to position ourselves to win the lottery rather than to be struck by lightning or to fall off a cliff. Perhaps we even think we are more successful at this game than, for example, an amoeba, yet it is clear we can be swallowed up ourselves or poke a hole in the aorta or be stuck by an HIV-contaminated needle no matter how many regulations OSHA prints.

In any case, I was thoughtful for about three months, after which I was told I should have a blood test to see if I had, in the kind of laconic fashion one likes to apply to these issues, "converted" and become HIV positive.

It turns out, of course, that I had not.

Still, these three months while I waited gave me something to contemplate on my off moments.

Who knows, now feeling lucky and in tune with the Strange Attractor, maybe I just might sally forth to the nearest 7–11 and buy a lottery ticket.

ORGANS, WHAT HO!

Heart time again?
I thought that was in February; but never mind, perhaps it is always "Heart Time." In any case I got something from some heart association begging that I give them a little more of my financial substance. I certainly will not and hope they will allow me to beg off, noting that I already sent them something in February, besides which my wife, lovely soul, also manages for some heart people, if not these, their annual drive for funds in our neighborhood.

As a result, nonetheless, of the superb efforts of those public relations firms which have "the Heart" as an account, I have been giving the matter of bodily organs a good deal of thought this past month, trying to determine which is my favorite.

I would be interested to hear from any of you who has your own particular answer to this question, giving your reasons for it, either scientific, poetical, or some combination thereof.

Look at it this way. Such a query seems a highly innocent pastime and if no great profit comes of such ponderings, so be it. At least it prevents me from thinking about all the regulatory agencies whose rules I am breaking daily, restoring somewhat my perspective as I return myself to that safe haven of considering our bodily organs. Besides, as I think of our organs, I tend toward the higher goal of perceiving thereby how alike indeed we all are as human creatures, despite the fact that some may tend toward being a bit more liverish or splenetic, big-hearted, brainy, or anally retentive (not that I am going to quite consider the anus an organ) as the case may be.

Perhaps, as well, I was stimulated to think organic thoughts as a result of a recent ad I saw in the paper, which indicated to me that the lawyers are beginning to do it, singling out certain organs and anatomical parts for specific legal attention and redress. The ad, surrounded by a broad, black band suitable for an obituary, busily impugned penile implants, and then went on to describe how the firm of Whomever and Whatnot, with an 800 number, was merrily seeking out gentlemen afflicted with a defective one. The date, hovering around April Fools' Day, stimulated my nurse, Mary, to concoct a scheme of calling said Whomever and Whatnot to set up an appointment for her husband, saying that he had had this surgery done and that the doctor had guaranteed that it would be absolutely safe and a little marvel of satisfaction. Waxing eloquent, she plotted a graphic description of how it had turned black and now was shriveled up, and was even more wee than it had ever been before, and that a piece of something that looked like plastic . . . "Oh, what if it was that terrible silicone!" . . . was sticking out from it. Of course, she would have finally said, "April Fool" to the 800 number, maybe, before hanging up.

I wander from the subject, and anyway am not sure that the male member needs to be dignified as an "organ" in the sense that I am meaning any more than the anus, even if some like D. H. Lawrence and Anonymous have called it such. Just as the skin is, in fact, the body's largest organ, regulating body temperature and trying to look good and all that sort of thing, I think I am not talking about these superficial sorts of "organs" that make big money for actors and ad agencies, but deep, dark organs lurking down in some hidden recess, smoldering away and doing their autonomic thing.

Let me return, therefore, to the heart. In brief, as I grow older, and therefore with more heartbeats in my past, approximately one zillion, I notice a perceptible augmentation of my respect for the heart. For many years, beginning even in medical school, I kind of sniffed at the heart, thinking it got more credit than it deserved. It seemed to me a rather stupid organ, doing nothing but pump. I discounted the poetry of this act altogether, and tried to pretend that it was merely fanciful that poets and those in love should feel the seat of their poetry and ardor to be located among all those *trabeculae carneae* and *chordae tendineae*.[1] In gross anatomy I never quite came to terms with where one circumflex vessel ended and the next began. I resented, for my own dark psychological reasons no doubt, all the publicity it got, its ability to make money, and the way beautiful ladies swooned at the sight of it. I am grown big enough now to admit my jealousy and my anger when, in the operating room for all those years after, I would ask in a quiet voice for a little straight-edged razor blade to take a tiny little graft for the skin's sake, and no one would ever know where such a two-bit instrument could be found. If I had yelled for the most advanced and phenomenally expensive cardiac whoop-de-do, it would have been produced immediately. For all these reasons and more I turned away from the heart, and sought elsewhere.

It was probably mere defiance and stubbornness, but for a long time I liked the spleen a lot. As an organ, it is such an underdog, a media non-spectacular, the liking of which possibly borders on affectation. Yet it was an unforgettable moment when I was first allowed to slide my hand down around the costal margin and feel the living spleen. I don't think anything compares to it for softness and smoothness. Besides, it is the organ acknowledged by both modern and ancient clinicians to be endowed with mystery, an organ I personally came to associate more with madness and the moon than any other, the *hysteros*[2] notwithstanding for these attributions.

---

[1] Rather odd ligamentous and muscular bands that line the interior depths of your heart, never demonstrated on valentines.

[2] That is to say the womb, or more anatomically correct perhaps, the uterus, thought to be a "wild" organ, which used to drive ladies quite crazy before the operation of hysterectomy was popularized. It comes directly to us as a reflection of these qualities in our use of the word "hysterical."

I am thus brought to the uterus, famous for provoking in ladies occasional fits of hysteria. I think it is not politically correct anymore to disparage the uterus for such associations, PMS excepted, unless the prostate is by some means equally belabored. For the record let me say that the prostate, unless enlarged and getting you up six times a night, or afflicted with cancer, does not even remotely command my attention as a "favorite" organ. The uterus, however, does. After all, what can be better than the veritable womb, within which hostelry you are treated to every luxury sufficient to cause any Ritz-Carlton to pale by comparison, and which, if you are a gynecological surgeon, is such a delight to take out, given due respect, of course, to the proper indications and bureaucratic oversight. The only thing I have never quite fathomed about this operation is why these ladies are always told they must not drive for six weeks.[3] What happens if you drive a car within six weeks of having your uterus removed? Surely you do not get hysterical or become more liable to a DUI, do you?

As for the liver, I reject it because it almost requires a PhD in organic chemistry to love it, and it is a very big nuisance when it takes to bleeding.

The lungs are too fluffy, and then sad when people turn them black through smoking. They become, indeed, tragic as they struggle on with life, heroically trying to trap a little oxygen and, in causing me to weep for them, forego, forgive me pulmonologists, the honors they deserve.

As for the brain, it always seems to me slightly unbelievable. As well, the brain is a little scary, not just because neuroanatomy was the very devil of a course, but because there is something suspicious about all those gyri and nuclei which, almost without your knowing it, may be up to something per-

---

[3] I have only recently been informed that were an accident to occur due to a lady's reluctance as a result of her surgery to mash hard enough on the brake she, you the surgeon, and anyone else standing around could be sued. I am glad, thirty years into my career, to finally have an answer to this question; which is a clear demonstration of how life is an ongoing learning process.

verse and maybe even wicked. In a science fiction movie I once saw there was a brain just like that, which had been taken out of some monstrous criminal and now lived in a fish tank full of brine, administered to by a mad scientist who, through this brain, gained hideous control over young ladies with beautiful skin and cleavage. It may sound like fun to have a spare brain like this on hand, but I could never go to such lengths, and will content myself to hope that I will simply live long enough until "virtual reality" will be in every home as a marginal substitute.

You have to admit, finally, that the skin is quite nice as an organ, if not afflicted by cystic acne and pustules. No one ever gives the skin much credit though, at least among the people I used to "run with," except to get irritated with it when they sunburned it. I always thought to myself, "Boy, if you were missing half your skin though, where then would you be? . . . and even if you were missing just a little piece of it, on some place noticeable, like your face, how would you get along at a cocktail party?" No one, even our professors in medical school, gave it much more than a passing glance for all its marvelous homeostatic capabilities and so on. For these reasons, skin appealed to me, besides which you could actually see it before your very eyes and maybe even do something with it. So I became a plastic surgeon.

Now, years later, even if I do not take it for granted, I am too much involved with it, and my perspective is too close to grant it a "favorite organ" status.

Accordingly, for reasons scientifico-poetical, historical, and marvellosal I have come home to the heart, the hearth that keeps within it the warm fire that lets us call our body "home," ticking and tocking night and day, rain or shine, through (we hope) dreams and nightmares, propelling us through life with an expenditure of energy which, if harnessed properly instead of being frittered away, would take us how many times, do they say, to the moon and back?

Heart, do you hear me? I pay you this compliment.

So just keep on rolling.

And maybe, come to think of it, I'll send you a little more money after all.

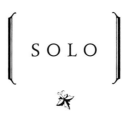

SOLO

I went to visit old *Tom Herbert the other day, that is, Tom Herbert,*
MD, pediatrician and character extraordinaire. As for being "old," I
use the adjective merely because he is 84 even though going on 60
years younger and requiring, when he blows off his back deck and
trims a hedge, a dash of extra oxygen in combination with a discreet ounce
of a better brandy.

His wife out on an errand, Tom let me in, looking for all the world perfectly fit, the only suspicious element being that at 4:00 in the afternoon he
was yet clad in his pajamas. But did they have a crease down the pant leg?
With his height, stature, and a stiff mustache reminiscent of something a
guardsman might sport, his pajamas signified a lot less of debility than of
comfort. By force of personality, Tom can make anything "look good," rather
like Churchill accomplished accoutered in a Siren Suit smoking a big cigar.

Tom ushered me into his back bedroom and sat down comfortably in his
chair. He had a stack of books on one side of it and a handsome bottle of
Very Superior Old Pale on the other. I noticed his oxygen machine, looking
a bit forlorn and even out of place, on the other side of the room. It had a
long plastic hose attached to it, which I assumed, whenever Tom took to
blowing off the deck just outside, he stuck up his nose and thus outfitted
made quick work of local tasks. Tom is that sort: Take it on, give it hell,
shake it like a dog a bone, drop it when the meat is gone, and go off to look
for more. He has been this way all his life; it is vaguely intimidating to us
merer mortals who have trouble finding bones at all.

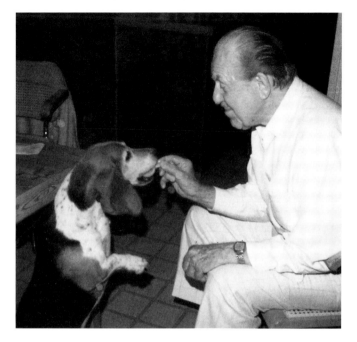

Dr. Tom Herbert and an anonymous dog.

Well, I was out there to pay my respects and so on. After all, sincere respects are indeed due anyone who, for 84 years, has been shaking bones and, to paraphrase Polonius, being to his own self so steadfastly true. I would dare say that Tom, unlike Polonius however, has probably made many a person and even patient quaver.

Tom is a quintessential old-school physician. Now we all wring our hands and kowtow, hope for the best, and beg our patients not to sue us. In his day, and I dare say even if he were practicing in our own, old Tom wouldn't give a damn. He would let 'em have it with both barrels; and if they took it or left it, it didn't matter to him. After all, he had done his duty. And he did, by golly!

Tom likes to consider himself as having been my pediatrician. I don't think he was, but he may have once looked at a sniffle in my dirty nose. Tom knew my family well, however, our clan having been modest fish relative to the tiny pond we lived in down in Mississippi County, Missouri, 30 miles south of Cape Girardeau, the hometown of Rush (Limbaugh), where in 1935 Tom set up his practice.

He was the first and only pediatrician between St. Louis and Memphis, and performed the first blood transfusion ever heard of on a child in swamp-east Missouri. Cape Girardeau at that time sported perhaps 15,000 or 20,000 souls, and pediatrics as a specialty had scarcely been heard of. Tom made his way by taking on obstetrics as an aside. It was through this obstetrical connection that he became acquainted with my family. Both Tom and my father were "gentlemen" of the same "old school." Although my father got along mostly on wit and charm, Tom added an enormous energy toward achievement. I always wonder from whence people get this latter, so I had dropped by for this visit, not only to pay my "respects" but to be instructed.

I gave him a bottle of pale sherry, which he may or may not drink because old school gentlemen sometimes consider this light stuff. In any case, after the initial ceremonious remarks, Tom and I settled down and had a damn good chat. He has strong opinions on everything, which adds to the fun.

By 1945, after he had returned to Cape Girardeau from World War II, Tom established himself firmly in a practice fully devoted to pediatrics, devising in the local schools a program for teaching what I guess were then called "the handicapped." He knew all about this subject for sure, and I was curious to hear him dead set against putting kids with Down's syndrome in regular classrooms. But Tom is what one would call an optimistic iconoclast. He doesn't want anyone to tell him how things ought to be done when he knows quite well himself how they damn well should be done, and there's an end on it.

In the last years of his practice he quit paying any kind of malpractice premiums, dropping that nonsense and telling folks they'd better be careful if they ever sued him. No one ever did, of course; he's not an easy target.

In the '80s he had had enough and retired to Tallahassee where he has been on hand as a bully philosopher ever since.

Tom told me he never had a partner because he "damn well didn't want anyone telling him what to do." I thought, for a brief moment, that maybe that was the way I felt too because I had (almost) never had a partner either. I thought to myself, "Ha! I am capable of strong convictions too, sufficiently firm in my self-possession that, therefore, I would not particularly put up with partners either." For a moment I basked in the prestige I had granted myself, but then doubt crept in, a disappointing, wheedling doubt, the kind of thing I am susceptible to, and which, just from the doubting in itself, made me see how thoroughly different I am from Tom, in spite of the strong image with which I had momentarily endowed myself.

It dawned on me that, contrary to his experience, my own reason for being in solo practice was not just because I didn't want anyone threatening to tell me what to do, but because I would have caved in, wrung my hands, and by all means done it, and then felt guilty in the aftermath for having so easily given up my own opinions to theirs. Yes, it was almost an insight; I am simply too susceptible to other points of view, their delicate nuances, their shades of intent and meaning. This is why con artists flock to me and I give them money, just like any little old lady and her cat.

But then, on the other hand, at least I have thus far survived being in solo practice. With Tom I take pleasure and pride, as might also all those other solo practitioners left alive, that we are a curious if dying breed. Never mind that Tom stayed solo because he did not want to put up with anyone else's opinion, and I have done so because I knew I would too much put up with them. He and I meet on at least tangentially equivalent terms.

In any case, having had this chat with Tom, I think I am going to dose myself with a dollop of sherry, or maybe even (for the weekend is upon us) start not being so capable of finding myself put upon. So there. What do you readers think of that?

Wait 'til you see me next time you meet me! Maybe I'll grow a bristling mustache! Maybe I'll even be four inches taller! Or some day, maybe, as tall as Tom.

THE NOSE KNOWS

I have lately been thinking, as I drive along, about the importance of inconsequentia. These musings involve an appreciation, more or less, of the fact that "It's the little things that count," the little folks that make history as much as the great heroes; how lice, and scabietic mites for example, have devastated more armies than cannons.

I suppose it is not altogether a *non sequitur* that I should think in the next breath about noses. If other physicians, while paused at a red light, think about more weighty matters, such as the Islets of Langerhans[1] and gastro-esophageal junctions, it seems to me I can allow myself a few thoughts on schnozzolas, a dated term, I believe, not heard since Jimmy Durante died.

I have the feeling that the nose has both made, or contributed to the not-making of, many men, and women too. How would de Gaulle have done with a little button nose like Doris Day? Little things sometimes count a lot. Would Hitler have been Hitler without his moustache? What plastic surgeon would dare change the nose of Meryl Streep or Barbra Streisand, and what will happen if one day a chunk of silicone extrudes from the nose of Michael Jackson?

The nose is a terribly important and subtle appendage. My own not being very great, I have accordingly always somewhat believed that a great nose (after all) is the sign of a great man; as for women I know not. No one has answers to such iffy questions, but just because there are no answers, as

---

[1]Spotty bits of glands within a gland, namely the pancreas, helpfully producing out endogenous insulin; in no way a vacation spot in the Caribbean visited by big red boats.

with so much else in life, it does not mean the effect is not expressed. Freud, of course, in his seminal study of the classic Wolfman Case, made the observation that the nose has something terribly important to do with the penis, another appendage great in mythology, about which I will allow the urologists their own due musings while waiting for the red light to change.

Unlike the plastic surgeons I read about in magazines, I have never done any famous noses; most of mine have been on ordinary people who see a disproportion stuck upon their face, or have been hit a good blow with, for example, a cue stick or a railroad tie, and in due course wanted it fixed. Even this category of patient, once sobered up a little, duly recognizes the fact that the nose is smack dab in the middle of the face and, for some strange reason, should be there without too gross an angulation. So we try to fix all of these things, for the good of mankind, with a subtle attention to detail that disallows simply another whack on the opposite side with the same blunt object.

I probably started reminiscing about noses I have known as a result of reviewing the literature on Tycho Brahe, the great 16th century Danish astronomer. He was an extravagant character, the "first watcher of the skies" to put calculations of stellar positions on a formal, computational basis, thus plunging us into the realm of modern observational technique. He had a streak of megalomania about him, and sensitivity too; in any case, taking light offense over something or other, in the subsequent duel he had his nose chopped off. He wore the defect with tremendous panache and cut—for his portrait image comes down to us—a rather dashing figure wearing a specially made silver nasal prosthesis (as a pirate might a black patch over a purportedly injured eye) to cover what is sometimes rudely called "the nose hole." Dressed all in inky black like Laurence Olivier in his great role as Hamlet, with a nice ruffle of lace about his neck and wrists, he was a striking image. But it was his silver nose, inlaid with gold, that sets him apart from the merely historically famous.

I have, of course, known a number of in absentia noses myself, one of which came complete on one of the most commanding personalities in local

Tallahassee society. When I knew this interesting lady, who owned most of our downtown, she was totally without nose, it having been eaten away by a basal-cell cancer. She was in her late 70s or so, and came to my office for a consultation. On this occasion she wore, as she ordinarily did when she went out, a complex paraphernalia of Band-Aids precariously constructed over the nasal aperture. At our first meeting I examined her closely and duly began to pronounce on the ancient Hindu method of reconstructing noses by turning down a forehead flap. Eloquently I described how the afflicted might thereby avoid the stigma associated with nasal absence in those woolly days when nasal amputation was a punishment of criminals, not only simple criminals but also adulterers, which meant that there were a lot of noseless people in 5th century B.C. India. I waxed on eloquently about the English surgeon Carpue who in 1816 first published his experience with two cases using this method to reconstruct noses, warming to my subject, and so on.

My patient, in due course, and in spite of my enthusiasm, interrupted me to say that she was only there for me to examine her feet. Cut short, I blushingly switched to her feet, upon which I found a variety of calluses which, *noblesse oblige*, she allowed me to pare down with nice aplomb and discretion. Nothing more was said about her nose, but to her dusty, albeit regal, eyrie on the top of the Hotel Floridan, where she had lived some 50 years of her life, I duly went a-calling whenever her calluses needed paring. Afterwards I was rewarded by a dish of sherry and small talk regarding her vast collection of antique Chinese snuff bottles. I learned from this experience that not everyone minds being without a nose, and that the physician should not jump to conclusions about what the patient may be consulting one about.

Perhaps my greatest nose job, even though it turned out to be a blob, was on Beatrice. Beatrice is the kind of "case" that usually happens to you immediately after your arrival in a community. Beatrice, whom we all came quite to love over the months (yes, months) she spent in the hospital, was inclined to spirits for her inspiration. When she arrived at the emergency room, no

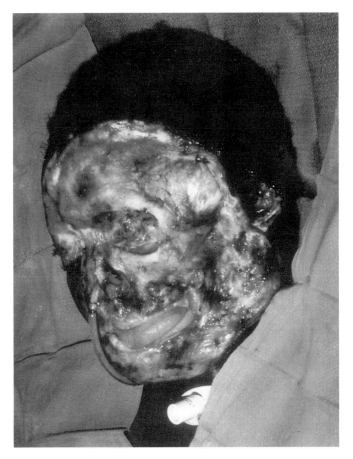

Beatrice—burned down and through the bones of her face.

one knows how many hours after her last drink, she had a blood alcohol level of 600 or so. At an earlier moment in the evening she had apparently passed out, her face inopportunely landing directly upon the burning, red hot coals of her open fireplace.

She is the only patient I have ever seen with an actual burn charring a bit of brain, penetrating right through the frontal bone. As a part of the initial debridement, I found it mildly appalling to find myself, with a neurosurgeon assisting, removing charred fragments of frontal lobe. Her face, eyes, and a good deal of the bone structure that we like to associate with one's features

74

were gone. But Beatrice quite merrily survived it all, and after tossing flaps about here and there, some of which lived, some of which died a bit, we finally were left with something that resembled a face, but no nose. I put up a great long flap, extending from her neck way down her arm, a sufficiency of it actually surviving so that Beatrice ended up with what vaguely looked like a muffin for a nose. But there it was!

She went home and, in the highest traditions of medical care restoring people to their former lives, steadfastly took up drinking again and died of a pulmonary embolus some three years later. But at least dogs did not bark at her, nor children throw stones, and when she sneezed—don't forget the benefits of a nose for this purpose, particularly in polite society—the force of the issue was discreetly directed downwards, far better than into the face of whomever you might be intimately talking with. By all means does the nose have its advantages.

On the other hand, of course, the external nose has extraordinarily little function. It is mostly social. It is awkward to go noseless to a party and enjoy polite conversation even with the most broad-minded party goers. People simply expect a nose in the middle of your face. And so, I beg you, forgive us plastic surgeons if we fiddle with the nose and think about it as I have been doing here.

There is more to it, thoughts as well as patients, but space forbids. Sufficient is the point that everything has its own wonderfully subtle importance, little though that iota may seem among greater and more flamboyant issues, but which in their effects make us all very much what we are. I wish I could be wiser about this.

Maybe I'll spend next month thinking about the silly appendix. There is no telling what devastations its rupture has caused throughout history. Never mind the inconvenience of postponing Edward VII's coronation in 1903, leaving a lot of Gurkhas, and all the other trappings of Empire brought to London at great expense, standing in the rain.

THE THREE GREATEST

In the last essay, I ended up threatening to reflect on the appendix. Why not? After all, to do so may be marginally better than leaving these pages blank.

For the present, however, and until policy is developed regarding blank page inserts in books and journals, I am going to flesh out these that are so graciously permitted me with something or other, and hope the appendix, like the nose, will disclose something somewhat more worthwhile than its contents of simple fecaliths.

Allow me, therefore, the latitude to say that as I pondered the appendix I came up with the insight, arguable perhaps to some, that the three greatest advances of the 20th century have been the result of discoveries, if not outright developments, made by physicians.

I was paused at a red light, congratulating myself on not having run the yellow, and thereby given the opportunity to do what I shall call "think." This is possibly the only moment in my day when I have time for "free thought," because otherwise I am continually either talking to patients on the telephone or in person, or taking off a wart, or letting our dogs and cats in and out through various doors.

As I drew breath at this red light, I thought how lucky I was. Oh, granted, it flashed through my mind that like anyone I take a great deal of pleasure in wringing my hands over the "temper of the times," the confusions, alarms, difficulties, stress and anxiety, the threats, taxes, and bureaucracy, the break-down of my '79 Toyota which must have the engine reamed out, the proliferation of acronymic agencies intent on our regulation, the medicolegal issue, silicone, the plight of the codfish on the Grand Banks, and so on.

All of this, and vastly more, swirls about us in confusing array, but I took comfort in recognizing that at least I am not living a prehistoric life as a hunter-gatherer, emerging fearfully from my dank, cold cave to try to bludgeon a rabbit or find a nut to bring home to my family. One of the great compensations of modern life is that probably none of us is going to be eaten by a saber-toothed tiger. Even the government is going to have to get a lot worse before I will be willing to trade in my present circumstance, with all of its stresses, for those that surrounded Cro-Magnon man and woman.

It was at this point that I thought how I should not even be here at this red light. I should have been dead 42 years ago when my appendix ruptured and, due to a bit of old-fashioned, house-calling misdiagnosis on the part of our curmudgeonly but naturally lovable family doctor, I was treated merely with high doses of laxatives. When I became anuric, and went vaguely off into a coma, it was decided that something was going on more than milk of magnesia was likely to correct, and that a dash of surgery might be in order. I was explored, Penrose drained, and given shots of penicillin and streptomycin. Without "torturing" the point whatsoever, I have to give Alexander Fleming, the discoverer of penicillin, a lot of credit and thanks, and I think you will have to allow, even if you disagree with my other choices, that antibiotics in this century have got to be a *summa cum laude* accomplishment.

In the middle of the red light by now, I still had plenty of time to lead myself on, for how can you let such a mighty thought process lapse without concluding an answer to the question, "What are the three greatest advances that have occurred in the 20th century?" These things, after all, must be rounded off, and Trinities seem to do it for us better than any other number.

My immediate response, beyond antibiotics, was Publix (or any good supermarket) and air-conditioning. These, I protest, represent the three greatest gifts given us in this century, although I am also willing to allow those north of the Mason-Dixon line, if it still exists, to substitute something else for air-conditioning. Otherwise, anything else you might care to name can go quite by the boards, including the airplane (contributes to anxiety), the telephone (to which we are enslaved, especially at dinner time), atomic energy (snuff us all out), the computer (see "2001" again), and certainly television (breeds violent couch-potatoes).

Consider Publix, if you will, and my case that it represents an unimaginable Utopia of foodstuffs, more conveniently packaged than manna from Heaven, a veritable apotheosis of huge varieties of comestibles efficiently delivered almost to our doorstep. The plethora astonishes, nor do you have to risk being eaten by a saber-toothed tiger to bring home not merely a nut, or a root, but such a selection of nuts and roots that would utterly bedazzle protoman, and for that matter a majority of folks in the world today. There is nothing that gives me a greater feeling of hope, progress, and well-being than going to Publix with my wife. Food, after all, is as important as health, and it is hard to imagine how it could ever be delivered better or more pleasantly.

In his first book, *A Thousand Mile Walk to the Gulf*, John Muir, the great naturalist, describes how in 1867 he walked through the South, traversing Florida between Fernandina Beach and Cedar Key, from thence taking a vessel to Cuba, and onwards to New York to deliver oranges. He notes that half of them were rotten by the time they got to their destination. I think of little kids in Victorian times, like Tiny Tim or the Little Match Girl, who would have been ever so happy to get an unrotten orange, considering it a marvel for Christmas. Our own daughters, jaded, would scorn an orange and be miserably disappointed, and even we veritable grown-ups are thoroughly, if deliciously, spoiled by the surfeit. No, I say, what more glorious, what more rapturous than Publix with its plenitude spilling at our footsies. Of all the things in our country the world might indeed envy, it is of this sort, computers and space shuttles a poor second.

And have we not, thought I, Dr. Pasteur to thank to some considerable degree for this capacity to maintain foods and beat back Rot? Why not? Permit me!

As for air-conditioning and the technology of refrigeration, which enhance our comfort and beat back rot to boot, we have another physician to thank, Dr. John Gorrie of little old Apalachicola, Florida, which is a mighty far place from the Pasteur Institute. Perhaps some may think that air-conditioning is a frivolous choice, even hedonistic, and not worthy of being included in the Great Triumvirate. As for myself, since those heady days when I first arrived in Florida in a black Porsche 911, un–air-conditioned, from New Hampshire, I rapidly decided that in the purchase of any car I would rather have the air-conditioner than the wheels. I remember still too well those non–air-conditioned nights of my southern youth, with the cotton fields abloomin' outside my room window and me within, apant in the suffocating heat, windows open to let in more heat, and possessed (as sometimes occurs in youth) by The Itch, that deadly dermatitis which had a life of its own, only barely beaten back by dabbing at it with those little tow-elettes containing sulfa of some sort. Except for a ruptured appendix, there is nothing worse than The Itch on a hot night.

I therefore celebrate that physician, Dr. Gorrie, who practiced just down the road from Tallahassee. In those days there was a big business bringing ice around from the New England states into the Gulf where it was packed into big sheds, and divvied out parsimoniously and at great expense for some social purpose or other. Dr. Gorrie, busily engaged in treating various tertian and quartan fevers on this malarial coast, developed empirically the not unreasonable idea that cooling the patient would assist in treating the disease. All by himself Dr. Gorrie invented a Rube Goldberg–type apparatus for achieving this purpose, a model of which can yet be seen in his house, now a museum to this great benefactor's memory. Of course the great new England ice cartel descended upon him *en masse* and beat his invention back,

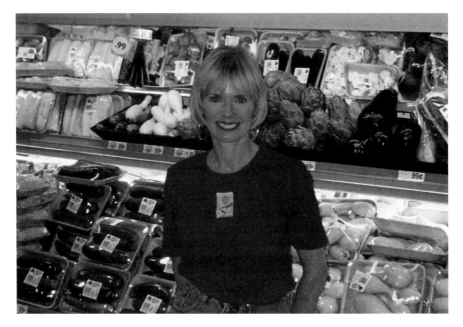

Lynn, whose husband I am, in front of some
squash, assorted artichokes, and a few eggplants, bless 'em!

not wanting their own economic circumstance threatened. It was really, I suppose, not until the 1930s that his invention began to be put to good use, in movie theaters mostly, where we thankfully went in the heat of summer. Look at it this way: The economic growth of the South took off once it became air-conditioned, so what can you say, never mind saying anything about trying to sleep and itch all at once.

Health! Comfort! Gastronomy! The Rise of the South! All of them the result of contributions made by physicians.

Suddenly I heard the honking of a horn, for the light had snuck its greenness up on me. Thrusting myself into gear I lurched ahead, and if there was a slight squeal of tires and a suspicious rattling beneath the hood, and oil leaking, the air-conditioner was working perfectly. Halfway down the block I pulled into the Publix parking lot, entered, and admired the varieties of pristine oranges, and lemons, and limes, and kumquats, and kiwis, and bokchoys all enticingly laid out. I paused sentimentally over the eggplants, for it was in Publix somewhere between the eggplants and the cabbages that I met the lady whom I got to marry and adore for the rest of my life. But I have become too jaded indeed for all these marvels. I passed them up and got some Shotgun Willie's "hot" salsa and a package of cholesterol-free dip-chips.

"Onwards and upwards," I said to myself.

There is nothing quite so nice as being alive in the air-conditioned comfort of Publix minus one's appendix.

WORKING (A LITTLE) FOR FOOD

It was a dark and stormy night . . .

But wait, I get ahead of myself. It may have been a dark and stormy night, but I was simply sitting around waiting for my beeper to go off, contemplating whether I could precipitate myself into the wild, wet, woolliness that was out there to fetch back from Hardee's a bunch of regular fries and some hamburgers.

And then it came.

The beeper tinkled, flashed, and vibrated. I dialed the number. Who was it?

Good heavens! It was his Right and Marvelous Honorableness Terry McCoy, MD, AMA Alternate Delegate; FMA Delegate from the Capital Medical Society; Chairman-Elect of the Medical Staff of Tallahassee Memorial Regional Medical Center; member of the Board, Health Plan Southeast; Vice-Speaker of the FMA (highly articulate, polished Irish tongue, etc.); past Member, FMA Board of Governors; past President, Capital Medical Society; President-Elect, Florida Medical Association; and Owner/President/Proprietor "Emerald Turf and Tree Sod Farms," and maybe "worms for sale" too. From his beautifully restored farmhouse-cottage 20 miles north, high up in Gadsden County, in spite of floods and drenching rains, he and his wife, Toni, were swimming on, doughtily entertaining guests at an elegant dinner party, never mind elemental forces.

Among the guests was also a child! And what's this? The child had fallen to strike precisely the point of his chin that kids like to strike, bursting it open. And here a bottle of the very finest wine was about to be uncorked

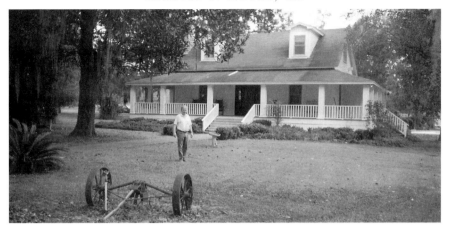

*Dr. McCoy strolling the grounds of his Gadsden County "estate,"
a great and succulent roast doubtless within.*

and a beautiful meal served actually at a table with chairs, knives, forks, etc., and even napkins. It was an emergency.

Quickly grasping the facts, I threw the cat in my lap to the floor, and sensing the urgency behind the calm, steadied tones of Terry's voice, said in reply, "Yes, yes, I see." And what's more, "I'll be there right away, through thick and thin," and so on; the intrepid plastic surgeon to the rescue over and across the flooded Ochlockonee!

I threw the cat again to the floor (this is a very persistent cat) and, gathering my family about me, namely, my wife, our 11-year-old daughter, and Maggie Mae, our greyhound, announced that we would have to set forth into the dusk and drive up into, can you believe it? the wilderness of Gadsden County.

I grabbed my syringes of Xylocaine, a length of nylon, my super-duper gold plated whooper-dooper needle holders, some gloves, and a box of Kleenex, and off we set into the wilderness and closing dusk. The clouds scudded across the raging horizon, their flaming colors, orange, pink, and purpura pregnant with meaning and rain. We were low on gas but pressed on. Crossing the Ochlockonee, its raging torrent heard beneath us, we turned left and went into the deeper bush, turning left again on an unnamed road that goes between somewhere and somewhere else. It was a wild and stormy night.

We passed through the great gates that flank the entrance to the long road leading to the McCoy Estate. And then, *mirabile dictu*, suddenly the lowering sky was opened and the setting sun's rays shone through like an almighty portent of auspicious circumstance. We let down the window so Maggie Mae could stick her long nose out. I could not help but notice how the wind blew my wife's hair into wild and random disarray, and the scent of her perfume flooded my nostrils. I gained control of myself. I stayed on the road dodging large puddles. The sun burst forth and I simply said: "And not by eastern windows only, When daylight comes, comes in the light; In front, the sun climbs slow, how slowly, But westward, look, the land is bright."

We pulled the car to a halt on the esplanade before the McCoy home. My wife got out and stood for an instant silhouetted in the glow of sunset, like Atlanta burning just over the horizon, her hair blowing once again. Should I sweep her into my arms like Rhett did in the poster? No, it would be too much like the wretched sequel, and my upper lip is too pale anyway, and, besides, we were here for more urgent purpose.

Anyway, I was saved from my fantasies by Terry and Toni and their son Robert emerging, greeting us, and leading us into the warm welcome of their charming home.

I put Rhett aside; now I was all Walter Mitty. It was older times, simpler times. There was a kitchen and a kitchen table. There was an overhead light. There was the little patient. A magnificent rib roast was just out of the oven, its aroma pervading my nostrils. But first, stifling all else, I did a quick but thorough examination. "It's a cut alright," I said tersely, "and it's almost a centimeter long, too." His pupils dilated, Terry asked, "Do you think it will take two stitches?"

My practiced eye saw immediately that it would be otherwise: "No, three," I said, with a confidence born of having already gone to the emergency room eight times so far this weekend.

We laid the little boy back while I numbed the area, my expert fingers playing over the wound deftly. There was a shriek, of course, but what can one say? We threw in the three sutures. Voilà! If only I were French, I would have said it!

Everyone was happy. We all danced. And then came the hard part. The McCoys, generous hosts to a fault, insisted that we stay for dinner and started shifting benches and boards into the dining room, dragging chairs about, and getting some place for Maggie Mae to sit. But we demurred. It was simply too much. We had to get back to our obligations before the river rose further.

We were just barely able to tear ourselves away; after all, we were not there to beg a meal.

We didn't need to. As we left, Toni, elegant, marvelous spirit, thrust into our hands, wrapped in a ton of tin foil, a huge slab of rib roast. We drove back only somewhat under 80 miles an hour because having this thing in the car was worse than being in the car with a box of Lindy's fried chicken. But chicken is handier: You can grab a leg and eat it at a red light. This was otherwise.

We got home and laid to. Great slices of superb roast, delicious in its juiciness, wolfing it down. We opened a bottle of our best and cheapest vin rouge and wolfed this down, more or less with it. We had a wonderful meal.

And so lives yet the "old-fashioned practice of medicine," food and hospitality for small service. My advice: If the McCoys ever call you for a sniffle, go see them; brave the torrents. In any case I am now going to write them, asking if they could arrange, particularly because Tuesday and Thursday nights are most convenient for us, to have small lacerations at their place on those evenings. We will look forward enormously to coming up and, even, will be quite happy to bring our own chairs to sit on.

And bring our dogs too.

And maybe our white cat.

TEACHING AND LEARNING FOOD

Give me credit. Not once in the more than several years I have been writing these essays have I succumbed to that greatest of platitudes and written that "time flies." Nor, worse, have I ever couched the expression all the more egregiously in (shudder!) Latin, as a late uncle of mine was used to doing, all too often and to our despair, when he would cry out about "*Tempus fugiting!*" Whether he wanted us to think of him as a scholar—he read a book a year—or a comedian, we never quite could fathom.

I am now, however, allowing myself the prerogative to write both in a single paragraph.

I promise I would not subject you to such an ordinary expression were it not for an extraordinary circumstance. After all, it is not so often that one's very own professor of plastic surgery, regarded by myself as a mentor *non pareil*, should retire. Unlike sometimes merer mortals, actors and actresses and politicians who seem every now and then to get a kick out of "retiring," then coming back to haunt us when they need a further dash of money or to be juiced up by a shot of popular acclaim, professors of surgery are made of sterner, steadier stuff.

In any case, Dr. Hal G. Bingham, Professor of Plastic Surgery for 10 years at the University of Missouri at Columbia and then for 20 at Shands Teaching Hospital, is simply not that sort. His retirement was accordingly a special event, duly noted with suitable fanfare by his faithful staff at the University of Florida, and complete with a retirement dinner, speeches, etc., all neatly orchestrated.

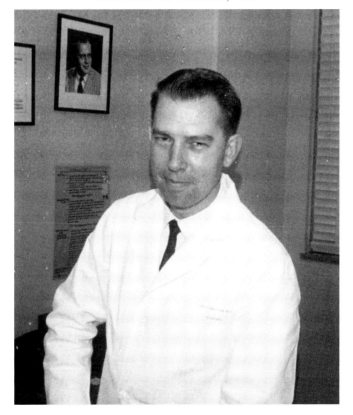

Dr. Bingham as I knew him then.

Having known Dr. Bingham and been mightily as well as happily influenced by him since I was a second year medical student on a three-week rotation to his service in 1962, I felt an appropriate chagrin that I was unable to attend the ceremonies that promoted him from professorship to some sort of vast, emeritus status. As my wife and I drove on the very day of his retirement dinner up to North Carolina to pick up our daughter, who had been at camp, I could not help but ponder the flight of these last 33 years since I first met Dr. Bingham.

I first met him over a cleft lip. As a haughty, supercilious, frightened, and callow medical student, I had been informed that I should present myself to the operating room at 8:00 A.M., and there stand in awe of Dr. Bingham while he did a repair of this lip. I was supposed to come equipped with a certain knowledge of the various techniques available to the plastic surgeon, and so had mused thoughtfully, surely late into the night, over books describing the various methods of reconstruction. I had made little sense of them. It seemed to me that there were a number of points like "A" and "B prime" and so on down the alphabet, all of them interspersed with terms like "advancement" and "rotation," which might have been clear enough if you were a ballerina, or in the description of folding a paper airplane, but to be performed on real flesh and blood seemed quite beyond likelihood.

I had arrived the morning of surgery a little paler than was my usual pallor as a second-year medical student, immersed in bacteriology and pathology, and had scrubbed according to the ritual we had been shown only a few days prior on our introductory perambulation of the OR suite. I had entered the room, my hands held up exactly as I had been taught ("Reach for the sky! This is a stick up!") to make sure that sterile water droplets ran downhill to my dirty elbows, rather than dirty elbow water dripping downwards onto my sterile hands. I felt absurd and intimidated by the drama of it all. Upon entering, I was immediately accosted by a nurse who told me I should tuck my shirt tail into my scrub pants . . . "I forgot". . . so germs would not fall from underneath my scrub shirt down into the child's mouth and wound. I was generally horrified that such "flora," as bacteria are rather whimsically and winsomely called, could tumble from my armpits, which, not being one of my favorite anatomical points anyway, I have always tried vaguely to suppress as even existing. I left the room, chastened, to tuck in my shirt and scrub again. I reentered, and was rushed brusquely into a gown and gloves and given a sterile towel to wrap about my hands in case some passing germ might nonchalantly decide to settle on my pristine purity. Like every medical and nursing student at such a time, you are walking on eggshells for sure.

The child was put to sleep. Dr. Bingham came in, curiously courtly in his manner, addressing me as "Dr. Moore," which almost made me light-headed.

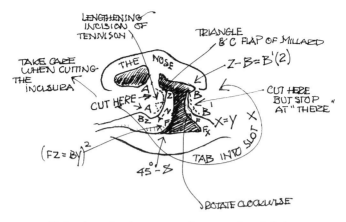

Medical student's version of repair of a cleft lip.

I watched him closely. I was like a duckling just out of its shell, ready to latch onto the first object I saw and follow it around and copy its every action forever. Thus the power of the teacher; for so, perhaps, I have done forever since exactly as Dr. Bingham did. I have always entered the operating room just so, taking care not to trip over a bucket, and sitting down graciously on a small, hard stool. Like Dr. B. I thumb through the chart and say something about the hemoglobin so as to demonstrate my command of laboratory values. Having done all of this himself, he left to scrub, returning it seemed to me in rather less than the ten minutes that had been drilled into us. Power, I supposed, had its prerogatives, even with germs.

We poised ourselves over the infant, I gaping at the hideous deformity, which in times past would have served quickly enough to leave a child exposed on a cruel hillside, or cast forth from society as a devil. Dr. Bingham called for the methylene blue and breaking a cotton applicator so as to achieve a nice point dipped it into the dye. Then, with a consummate grace and decorum, as though he might have been offering me an ice cream cone, said, "Dr. Moore, would you please make the marks for the repair."

Never mind that I was thoroughly appalled! I made a few passes with the methylene blue, which dried on the stick and would not make a dot at all. I wet it again and most tentatively hazarded a dot, which immediately, due to a small bit of saline still moistening the skin, diffused over the whole lip, making a great blob of blue. The nurse rolled her eyes at me, for she was cool and hard and beautifully experienced in her slightly cynical disregard for medical students. "Blue Blobs" never wipe off, no matter what the means and effort, if made by a second-year medical student. I made certain remarks barely audible and wrestled with the philtral margins, hoping I could bear them down anyway, and force from them a point that could be called the peak of a "Cupid's Bow." Gradually a series of rather randomly placed A's and A primes made themselves apparent; but was this the "A" or the "A prime" that went with the Lemesurier or the Tennison repair? I had mixed them up. And what about the new-fangled Millard and the "C flap" located somewhere or other? It all blended into one image. No sense could be made of it.

Dr. Bingham asked me a few questions, posed as always with the forbearance that defines a gentleman, and deftly cleansing away the mess I had made with a bit of alcohol on a sponge, carefully dried everything off, broke a new point, and called for his calipers. He then made immaculate measurements with all the proper points of prime and prime squared and logs of prime and primes plus "X" and "Y," connecting these with little lines. And there it was.

The cuts were made, the flaps lifted, rotations done, advancements performed, and, yes, before my callow eyes was a lip that God, having failed quite to make, had contrived through Dr. Bingham to be corrected otherwise.

During those three weeks, the techniques I was exposed to fashioned me profoundly, and things became a bit more clear. What became more clear than anything else was the clarity of Dr. Bingham himself. The straightforwardness, the integrity, the courtesy, the curious charm, the ease of manner, the confidence, the knowledge, the interest in his students, the care for his patients, that have stayed with me ever since, duckling that

I was, and remain now, 33 years later, an integral part of my own practice, I hope and think.

But of all the things he taught me the greatest lesson was to care about what we have been privileged to learn to do, and to show the patient that we care, and are aware that it is indeed a privilege. I like to think it was my best learned lesson from Dr. B. and that I, as merely one resident of his many, carry his endowment to us into the future.

His last residents will continue to do so for another 30 years or more.

Perhaps it is in a different sense than Hippocrates meant it, but indeed "Art is long," if "Life is short" and—begging your pardon again and with a "nod" to my Uncle Tom—*tempus fugit*.

REFUTIN' NEWTON

I was looking at our cat Dewey the other day and was reminded to be impressed, once again, by the manifold marvel of God's work. It does not matter whether your perception of God is from the far fundamental end of the spectrum or on the far metaphorical abstract. A cat is a wondrous work of imaginative creation.

My gaze turned fondly from Dewey to Maggie Mae, our "retired" greyhound as she lay elegantly balanced on her veritable spine, her legs sticking straight up in the air in a position you would think no greyhound could possibly contrive. I marveled at the exquisite definition of her toes and the elegant length of her nose. Then, hard by, was Buttercup, the miniature poodle, quite uncut and, therefore, looking round as a tub with pink bows at each ear, a tongue to match, and beyond anyone in the house, by far, knowing herself to be a ravishing beauty. This is quite in contrast to old Wick, our now quite blind and arthritic Yorkshire terrier, yet a gentleman still capable of spending a night out barking at a possum beneath our house and who, with his hair so oddly cut and his joints sticking out, looks a most magnificent artifact.

There we have it! Right at my feet were veritable wonders of creation. What if someone had asked any of us, starting from scratch with no precedents whatsoever in the entire universe to draw upon, to sit down at our drawing board and knock off a few million of nature's various flora and fauna. Each of everything is so much the same and yet so remarkably different. I merely look at Dewey, and beyond admiring him as a creation must go

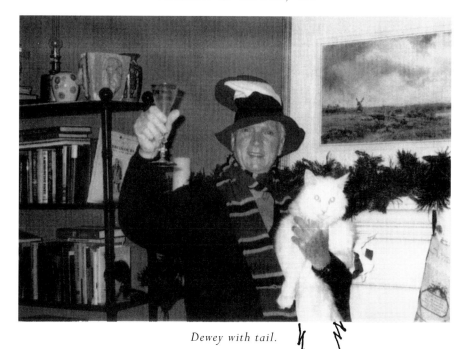

Dewey with tail.

a step further to find myself further charmed by God's great wit, which (for example) having knocked off the "Cat" in all its myriad and interesting forms including the Manx, and the Maine Coon, and the Curly Coated Rex, He could have gone on from there, having found the cat "good," to create the rabbit by a mere amputation of the tail, elongation of the ears, and substitution of "hoppers" for hind legs.

It is all such a rich and brilliant work. Even if the remark has been made before, surely there is no harm in making it again: Indeed, even to exclaim, "Lo, manifold are the works of God, and they are good!"

But even God, as I noted previously in my discussion of Dr. Bingham's repair of a cleft lip, is seemingly not perfect. Cleft lips and far worse also abound. We live, furthermore, in a world burdened by gravity, causing our steps to be heavy and, even worse alack! our tissues to sag. Above our heads, particularly in South Florida, burns that great cobalt unit in the sky that, though it might produce a handsome tan for those who can get a handsome tan, nevertheless nastily destroys elastic fibers in the skin, no more ever again to be created anew than brain cells accidentally slurped away by a neurosurgeon's sucker. We live in a world in which it was once fashionable to be seen smoking (amazing fact!), sucking noxious tars and ash into our lily-pink lungs, there to be transmitted by the least delicate capillary to every remotest cell, including the struggling skin. And finally, of course, we still live, despite quarks and all the other cosmological advances, in a mere Newtonian world where time, working hand in hand with gravity, drags us down, and we begin, for Heaven's sake, to look not like the wondrous selves we once were but more like, all of a sudden, our great, great grandmothers.

I believe you have caught my drift. Let me beg of you accordingly to catch it in a little wider sense. I am about to say that God has mercifully arranged, in all the vastness of creation, to give us also the expedients through which we may, with a little imagination of our own, cast even perhaps in God's image, remedy a few of the accidents and built-in ills that any vast structure, such as a universe, is bound to experience. Perhaps such is a large part of our happiest meaning.

Certainly I would like to suggest, in humble fashion, that such is a part of the physician's very particular privilege. Every one of us, even the homely plastic surgeon, experiences every day some small (or is it all that small after all?) event that suggests we are more than we sometimes think.

I had the pleasant experience, experienced equally by other plastic surgeons and I would guess perhaps even more so by other physicians in other fields, of just such an occurrence. A lady very pleasantly telephoned me from Virginia a couple of months ago. In 1978 I had fixed her nose with a bit of a rhinoplasty and had put in a little chin implant. In 1979 I had done a facelift and blepharoplasty when she was age 51. She now wanted a repeat facelift after these 16 years of ongoing gravity, and so flew to Tallahassee to allow me to perform this procedure. During the course of her visit, she informed me of the good meaning of her surgeries undergone in the late '70s. Far from, as is sometimes suggested, being mere frivolous "vanities," she described how they had given her such a renewed sense of confidence that she had, scarcely dreaming she could win the award, applied to Smith College for a scholarship to obtain her degree. She got the scholarship, quit her secretarial job, packed her cat and gear in her car, and sallied forth to graduate four years later, *summa cum laude*. She now has a highly responsible position at a well-known college in Virginia. She generously, and with obvious sincerity, ascribes to the surgeries I performed her capacity to have embarked on this happy career, which even now she marvels at having accomplished.

That we should participate in people's lives with such direct effect is a pleasure much to be valued.

Perhaps it is a characteristic of growing years living in a sagging Newtonian world that such awarenesses become more appreciated. Similarly, a fine glass of modest wine or even a martini can be better savored than when I was 25. So too I can better marvel at the small tufts of hair that stick out from between Dewey's toes; the exquisite definition of Maggie Mae's muscle structure combined with her delicacy of bone, of Buttercup's most wonderfully self-assured sense of her own beauty and worth, and Wickie's fierce but scruffy terrier self, though blind, defending his hearth and home from all possums.

Forgive me if in "The Good, the Bad, and the Homely" you might not expect to be reading a sermon. The mind also probably succumbs to a bit of Newtonian gravity; the pity being that the neurosurgeons cannot give our brains a nice little "lift."

Oh well, maybe I'll get someone to do me a little "tuck" about my jowls, call it "sweet" if temporary "revenge," and see if my brain will consider applying for a scholarship at Smith.

EVERYTHING, AND MORE, I KNOW ABOUT X-RAYS

Truthfully, I have never had any personal associations with Röntgen or the Curies, Madame and her husband.

The nearest I have come is taking a certain pride in remembering how to spell Röntgen's name, and in baby-sitting a big brindled cat who lives across the street from us. Her name is Curie.

It is an odd name for a cat. On the other hand our charming neighbors who own her are a little odd themselves. He is Australian, but of a different sort than "Crocodile Dundee." Her mom was a French intellectual and her dad a professor. They are much more intellectually inclined than anyone else on our street, so it is hard, often enough, to fully understand them.

In any case they have very bright children, and just prior to achieving[1] this cat, which (being intellectuals) they thought was the thing to do because every other regular family on the street has a cat, they had *en famille* watched the film "Madame Curie," I think starring Paul Muni and Greer Garson. The "exposure" was something of a teaching exercise, so they overlooked the

---

[1] The use of this word, for this purpose, has caused hot debate! There are those sufficiently unfamiliar with the beauty of the feline mind and psyche as to suggest that the word should have been "acquired." But no one, I herewith remonstrate, who knows to admire the mind of the cat, could ever think of them in an acquisitional sense, as you might think of, say, a Jackson Pollock painting. "Achieve" is patently the correct choice of word, not should it be compromised by being placed in anything so mundane as quotation marks. Accordingly, it is with gratitude, and a deep faith in the impeccable sensitivity of her judgment, that I wish to thank the copy editor of this work, Carol Field, who struck upon an acceptable solution, breaking what had become an impossible impasse, by suggesting that we apply a footnote to the issue.

harsh fact that the movie was not even in color. The elevating effect upon the children was to name the cat Curie, which is, as I have perhaps implied, quite a lot to name a cat.

Curie, as it turns out, is no intellectual but likes to fight. She spends much time over at our house with her claws unsheathed, rendering havoc among our own happy animals and ourselves. Even so, we took her on, introducing her to the very lap of luxury in our very own home for the entire summer while the intellectuals were away for two months on Cape Cod, basking and intellectualizing. Gradually, as the summer wore on, Curie calmed down slightly, drawing less blood, soothed by our commonplace intelligences and the superb cuisine.

That, for the record, is the totality of my experience with Röntgens and Curies.

I am, however, a tremendous admirer of the x-ray apparatus in general. What better, more marvelous bit of science might we find to blame for having launched us into the miracle of modern medical technology? True, there is the thermometer, which by the turn of the century had been around for 50 years or so but tended to get nowhere; and maybe Einthoven's prototype of the cardiogram was on the verge of making its squiggle; and perhaps some advanced clinician was even by the turn of the century taking a blood pressure now and again, marveling. But such prosaic little apparati pale in comparison to capturing the Röntgen ray.

Within a matter of months after its introduction 100 years ago, the ray had been applied to the diagnosis of disease in Egyptian mummies, and we learned that high priests had no osteoarthritis, whereas the workers and dung beetles, who pushed sand blocks up the great pyramids, had a lot of it. Pretty soon children, I myself indeed, could stand in shoe stores and see the bones of our feet right through our leather shoes, green and eerie with lots of beta particles. Pretty soon after that we had the CAT scan, an ingenious marvel almost equal to the cat itself.

Truly, as I see it, more than anything else, x-rays represent the real magic of modern medicine. But they also required real magicians who sprang up in the form of what we now call radiologists, who, with great daring risk their own and even their progeny's lives, braving lymphoma and fingers falling off and coffee addiction. In compensation they possess the happy knowledge that they are a part of that select few, that happy, happy few, who have perhaps more than any group of medical specialists led us out of darkness and upwards into those broad pastures of utmost medical technology and extravaganza of cost. They are part of that honored breed defining specialization at its acme. Who now would dare have a headache without a CAT scan to go with it?

For what it is worth, I take great pride in noting that I, too, once operated a real x-ray machine, almost all by myself. When I was the lonely little solo doctor-surgeon at the little old mission hospital in Namitete, Malawi, just out of my internship more or less in the mid-60s, I was confronted often enough with perplexing, I-don't-know-what-to-do kinds of circumstances. The mission hospital was run by some French, Austrian, and Alsatian nursing sisters, a right jolly, pink-cheeked bunch, who knew mostly what to do. But from time to time they were at a loss themselves, as was I. They had inherited from one of Rommel's panzer divisions a trunkful of surgical instruments, a library of medical books all in German hopelessly describing mostly German diseases (judging from the pictures), and a field x-ray unit that folded up so it could be conveniently carried in a tank. When I didn't know what to do, I would always bide for time by saying "Let's take an x-ray!"

We would then unlimber this apparatus and put it on its tripod of legs, constructing a delicately balanced configuration that looked very much like a flamingo standing on one leg. Some knobs would then be turned, as I recall, and the beak pointed at the place that hurt. Rather like Dr. Frankenstein, we would then gather together a jolt of electricity, and push a button, and wonder if anything had happened.

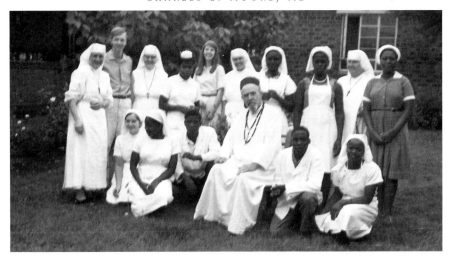

The staff, the Mission Hospital, Namitete, Malawi, 1967.

One of the sisters actually knew how to develop the plate, and disappearing behind a vaguely closed door would come out with the production sometime later. It would either show nothing or just a wee bit of something. It mostly, as I remember, showed "gas." If the abdomen had reached the size of a meteorological weather balloon I would then say, "We have to operate!" We would break open a can of ether, and do so, the rain beating down on the tin roof just like in Somerset Maugham. I would put a little tube into the billowing bowel and let everything decompress, hoping more or less that the patient would be alive the next day. It was amazing how often this worked!

Once we took a picture of a gentleman's chest, a sporting middle-aged German character sauntering through East Africa heading south, and I could just barely see that the heart was pushed way over into his right arm. I told him, not knowing what else to say, that he had a pleural mesothelioma and probably some TB too, and drew out about 20 liters of fluid from his thoracic cavity. We sent him by ox cart some 40 miles down the road to Lilongwe for treatment in an institution with slightly higher voltage. I often wonder, in the night, whatever became of him. Lilongwe, of course, was later made the capital of Malawi, and did all right.

So there you have it! X-rays, not to mention Lilongwe, have come a long way, even in my own lifetime. I marvel at where they will ultimately take us; and think it will be to that refined point where, like "Bones" in Star Trek, we can simply wave a little hand-held MRI-CAT-Scanner-Cobalt-Unit-Combo (the MCSCUC) in the general direction of the patient and find out everything there is to be known, including, of course, the sperm count and IQ.

What a convenience it will be! And surely cost-effective, too!

So, I say, all honor to Dr. Röntgen, the Curies, and our radiologist friends who have given us so much, and at some cost to themselves!

Yes, I am inspired by their example, and think I will go and rent the movie myself.

Perhaps we can even get a new cat: a good, tough tabby to defend us from Curie. After all, Röntgen would be a nice name for a cat, not forgetting the umlaut, of course.

WITH A FIFTH OF LAGAVULIN

In the last two months two new characters have walked onto the small stage of my life's drama.

Well, to be technically correct only one actually "walked on," young Dr. Colin Jamieson, a bonny braw Scots laddie about to qualify at the University of Manchester in England.

The other appeared more or less fully blown, not quite I think from the head of Zeus but at least fully armed. This is an entity heretofore utterly unknown to me called "Beech Street."

Young Dr. Jamieson, with his personal charm, winning manner, love of music and gourmet Scottish (sic) cuisine, and Beech Street, which is neither a person, nor an address, nor the title of a sitcom but some new layer of the medico-economic bureaucracy, have little in common.

Each, however, has nudged along my thought process about the "business" of medicine.

Colin arrived to spend six weeks with me on a "rotation" from the University of Manchester. I like to beguile my local colleagues into thinking that he came as a result of my international reputation, my skill and expertise in the practice of plastic surgery, the spread of my reputation beyond Sopchoppy and the Shores of Apalachee Bay, beyond Attapulgus, Georgia, even beyond Georgia, and lo! as far afield as the British Isles. It became clear that no one would accept this fantasy; so in the event I had to confess that I was approached by Colin's first cousin, who lives in Tallahassee, and who told me that Colin's curriculum insisted that he go somewhere for six weeks to see other methods and means, and that Colin didn't have any money to go almost anywhere at all. Accordingly he was coming to Tallahassee where his cousin would put him up on the cheap. When this plan came up months and months ago, it seemed sufficiently distant in the bland future that I glibly stated I would be glad to shepherd him about. It crossed my mind to wonder what in the world I would show him, and that he would get bored watching me take off follicular cysts and so forth; but such concerns were too far in the future to worry about.

It concerned me, too, that he might be some sort of classic, dour Scotsman, arriving dirked and sporraned, with a full set of bagpipes. I remembered the late famous actor, Richard Todd, in that film with Ronald Reagan, "The Lonely Heart," about a Scots soldier who never spoke a word to anyone; and hoped for the best.

Actually, "the best" was what I got. No one could have been easier, more affable, more bright and agreeable than Colin. He rolled his r's magnificently, and the young ladies I foisted upon him fell madly in love and tried to take him to the beach. He brought me a can of Scotland's finest haggis, and I fed him grits, and at his recommendation bought the most expensive bottle of Scotch in the entire world, which he said he always gave his dad for Christmas. We had a wee thimbleful, and a marvelous time.

I thought, of course, it might be "educational" to introduce him to the vagaries and complexities of our unique schemes for paying physicians for their services, while at the same time keeping down, *grace à dieu*, costs!

And here is where this entity "Beech Street" entered onstage. At the outset of our discussions respecting "medical economics," the British National Health Services was introduced as a positive model by Colin. I proffered him in return a slightly condescending smile. Coincidental with his visit, as we began studying the fine print of our own "Beech Street" contract hoping to determine what lay within and beyond, we (my office manager and I) worked ourselves up into a fine post-modern-payment-schemes-all-American frenzy.

"And what is this Beech Street?" asked Colin, with a fine roll to the r as always.

"Why," I riposted, "it is simply an intermediate organization, acting with the state, for the sake of the insurance company, in the name of the patient to provide, in due course, if the computers are running, recompense to the doctor, for caring for the patient, if the necessary administrative bureaucrat deems that the conditions have been acceptable within the terms of the originally signed contract between said doctor and the Beech Street entity."

"Oh," said Colin.

"We are," I said hopefully, "trying to keep what we call 'costs' down."

I left it at that. But the camel's nose was in the tent. Indeed, at this point, the entire camel stalked on stage, and . . . Colin, being a good chap . . . I broke down, just barely repressing my sobs, rending the air over the absurdity of what patients and doctors are being put through in this country. I even confessed that any slight condescension I had implied formerly towards his NHS was rapidly evaporating, and that our nation's means of paying its physicians seemed to be developing into a system designed for the worst of all possible worlds; becoming ever more a nightmare of increasing complexity wherein viciously vying health maintenance organizations, the government, insurance companies, and these new paying entities, like Beech Street, with whom we must sign further contracts, were put in place simply to torture us all. I noted, bewildered, how in the name of cost containment payments to doctors had tumbled, so that many could barely meet their overheads; and how, paradoxically, the premiums patients and ourselves were now paying annually soared precipitously. I hinted darkly that in the name of "cost-containment" huge chunks of money were being siphoned from both patients and physicians to go to vast new bureaucracies, seemingly invented overnight for the purpose of paying handsome salaries to administrators sitting behind desks looking at a world of clouds from the 34th story of large buildings thrown up for the purpose of seating them. I sobbed over the complexities of filing a claim, or trying to get an answer when you are constantly put on hold, and being told inevitably by an automatic voice to push other buttons . . . and so on.

Poor Colin was astonished. He is not used to the spectacle of seeing his mentors hysterical and in tears. He generously noted that the National Health Service had its disadvantages, but with private health supplementing it in rational fashion all seemed to run very smoothly from his perspective. He softly rolled a few r's at me, in comforting fashion. We had a peanut butter and jelly sandwich, and a glass of milk, which he knew would help me recover my equipoise, so sadly lost.

We are now about to sign a contract with someone, Beech Street or one of the others, and I have no idea what will come of it. I'm simply keeping my fingers crossed.

Colin has flown back home confirmed in the advantages of his system, but having had a marvelous visit to Tallahassee, I do hope. As for myself I am nudged, as I said, towards what is the contemplation of any insurance circumstance, almost, other than what we are developing.

Even a bit of some National Health Plan.

Well, perhaps, preceded by a fortifying wee dram of that finest Scotch.

GALEN LIVES!

There is nothing like experience, but learning a little something from it is not as simple as it sounds. Good for Galen accordingly! After all, there are usually plenty of (pretty good) reasons to suppress anything that might be learned from this and that. Sometimes one simply doesn't want to learn anything because one is so happy to be reasonably ignorant. A certain degree of ignorance, particularly when it is reasonably successful, has made you a bit of an income, provided some security and a roof over your head, dogs, cats, and an occasional vacation, food in the mouths of your children, (let me not mention their education) obviously works too well to tamper with altogether too much. Let well enough, indeed, alone!

But sometimes one does glean something from a bit of an experience. Sometimes things happen, if only idiosyncratically, that force us, at least me, to give a second look at a hitherto firmly held belief. I am not talking epiphany but just a wee gleam of insight.

Having had my necrotic femoral heads and hip joints conveniently replaced awhile back, I am now entertaining the likelihood of having my knee joints reamed out. As I contemplate the former orthopedic experience, looking forward to the future, I ask myself "what was the best thing about that experience?"

The unequivocal answer is . . . the blood loss!

Ever since medical school I have slightly sniffed, sometimes even scorned, the absurdities and "lack of knowledge" of medicine's "dark ages" when legions of physicians, starting with Galen, bled patients half to death in the name of balancing up their humours.

We all know about George Washington and his being quite bled to death by his learned physicians. We know about Lord Byron at Missolonghi and how he was bled white and languid, which he may have rather enjoyed, by Drs. Francesco Bruno and Julius Milligen, his two medical attendants. We know of the almost obsessive-compulsive passion with which the great American physician, and author of an enlightened treatise on *Medical Inquiries and Observations Upon the Diseases of the Mind*, Benjamin Rush, bled his patients. These men were all of good education and intelligence and must have perceived a meaningful benefit from their copious blood letting. We are no brighter, but tend to be condescending towards their practices.

Well, my own experience has led me to the belief that a good, nice, blood-letting would probably be a marvelous thing to do to lots of people, merely on general principle.

Following the removal of my two hips, and the lowering of my hemoglobin to about seven, I never felt more beneficently towards the human race; never so balanced with the universe and its great turnings. The music of the spheres was within my ken; I felt the most benignant sort of lassitude, and a certain knowledge that all would be "all right." For about three or four weeks, as I built my blood count up to a more usually frenzied plethora, I simply sat around turning the pages of picture books, admiring the art, reading a word or two, and blandly looking at the wallpaper. Everything was full of mystical meaning. As I look back upon it now, I can almost convince myself that a bilateral hipectomy by Dr. Dewey (after whom we named our second to newest cat) about every couple of months or so would keep me in a state of pleasant calm.

It is this fact, I believe, that Galen stumbled upon, cleverly recognized, and which physicians ever after until just recently embraced with enthusiasm. At last, they had something beneficial to offer their patients. After all, they had nothing otherwise except dull stuff like "fresh air" and "good diet" as recommended by Aesculapius. So why not draw a couple of pints of blood, or three, or even four depending on the circumstances? Why not formalize and codify into "Natural philosophy" the ancient wisdom of Earth, Air, Water, and Fire, getting those elemental primordia balanced in the blood.

Now the physician could enter the sick-chamber, marvelously hold up to the light a glass of urine, and, wrapped in the dignity of his robes, announce the science of black and yellow bile, phlegm, and blood. Then, awe inspiring in the act, draw off two or three pints before the patient's very eyes. The gleaming scalpel, the vein standing out blue and succulent, the deft flick of the lancet, a rich gushing and not even a drop on the floor! It all conspired to affirm both art and knowledge.

I can imagine the occasional lady, or more likely gentleman, fainting, servants running this way and that fetching hot water, the patient's eyelids fluttering. She has been in such a frenzy, after all. What is she sick with? Who knows? It didn't particularly have to matter, I think. The blood is so red. It is like something that would flow from Snow White. The basin gleams as it fills. There! It is done! It is worth, almost, a bit of applause.

And the patients? How marvelous they now feel. What a delicious languor pervades their every cell. How they fall back, and turn the pages of their book, if they have one, glancing at the pictures, if there are any, feeling nothing but lightheaded and marvelous. What is there to worry about? Nothing anymore. Everything has been put in its proper balance. All those vile anxieties are drawn out and a delicious weakness takes their place, which may include a regimen of frequent naps, and a pleasant tidbit of food. All is well with oneself and the universe, and if it isn't . . .

Well, the physician can always come back a while later and draw out another pint of blood. At some point, for sure, the patient will succumb to the euphoria of his or her anemia, which not only will feel good, but will be surely noted by all around as a kind of romantic other-worldliness. It is indeed, a thought.

As therapies go, in the absence of better, it doesn't seem so bad. On the other hand, speaking of outmoded therapeutics, I wouldn't mind pondering the resurrection, either, of long, languid sea voyages. (Keeping the waves, of course, under three feet!)

But possessed, in this case, by a hemoglobin of at least 12. After all, one likes to be in possession of at least a little energy when the band strikes up.

{ UNIVERSAL UNTRUTH BE DAMNED }

I cannot guess about you (of course!), but if I am called to the emergency room in the wee hours of the night, getting home at 2:30 flushed with adrenalin, my pupils dilated, my heart wildly pumping, my spleen jumping, and my bone marrow sloshing in my bilges, I need a bit of winding down.

Not that I am not immediately comforted by the sight of home, happy home! I love pulling into our driveway, getting out in the quiet night of our tiny neighborhood, and seeing a great moon floating through the dark branches of the two live oaks in front of our house. Indoors, I take a swig of skim milk directly from the plastic gallon jug (it tastes better that way, flavored by the surreptitious nature of the moment), pleasantly free from the chidings of our 12-year-old[1] who, perhaps with a little justification, finds the practice "disgusting."

This should compose me, one would think, for bed.

But no, the juices yet flow, and besides, how wonderful to be home to relish the peace and quiet. What to do?

I wonder mildly what most other doctors do? I wonder if there are patterns of recuperation in such moments preferred by certain species of physicians? It is hard for me to imagine what Tom Bixler, our heart transplant surgeon, does. For some reason I have it in my mind that Bill Long,

---

[1] I confess that recently I have caught her doing the same thing and chided her myself! Which brings up the question regarding whether this is an inherited or learned trait.

one of our well-known vascular surgeons, reads a book on cosmology. I think urologists do something both fun and funny. Orthopods probably go out and chop wood by the light of the silvery moon and sing ribald songs. Shrinks may write poems or do kinky things. I like to think that Jesse Judelle, internist and aviator, simulates flight on his computer. Perhaps I like to think that because it is one of the things I enjoy doing myself at such a moment, and I admire Dr. Judelle quite particularly.

One of the reasons, a minor one but true nevertheless, that I still go to the emergency room when I could have "retired" from that sometimes onerous chore a few years back, is because I have a kind of nostalgic pleasure for these moments when, the case over and done with, I get to return home to that moment. Beyond that, these fragments of nocturnal privacy have actually taught me something not only vaguely about myself, but also, I am almost willing to say, a great truth about our place in the universe, namely, that we can learn things in spite of ourselves.

After all, it has been in these small-hour moments that I have learned to work our computer, and if this contraption is not a "Great Universal Truth," a kind of electronic microcosm of the universe, I know not what else it may be.

I got into the computer via, I confess, a game. But it was not just any old game, it was "Jet Fighter II." It was a few years ago when my wife gave me this game. She remembered a little snapshot taken of me when I was about eight sitting in front of a cardboard "instrument panel" wearing a little helmet and goggles, pretending I was piloting a P-40 in the early days of World War II. I spent almost the entirety of that war flying missions for the allies, pretending I was "Dave Dawson at Dunkirk." I was ultimately serious enough about all of this so that after college I went by way of the NROTC to Pensacola to begin flight training; wretchedly, but in my case probably lifesavingly, some cold, calculating, insensitive, unyielding, ophthalmological flight surgeon who rechecked my eyes about four months into the course, using an overdose of atropine, threw me out and into the fleet. I pouted and decided I would never fly again; and did not until the computer and "Jet Fighter II" came along. Now I can land on carriers blindfolded with my hands tied behind my back. Thus do I go to bed, my catecholamines depleted after a few successful missions.

More important, as a "Universal Truth," it has been at this moment of the night that I have discovered that you do not have to be born with a "musical ear" to learn a bit of music. More than jet fighter, the piano has become my happiest physical means of relieving pressures and pent-up emotion. I am not speaking Chopin Nocturnes, by the way, not at all. But I have discovered what I think music teachers refrain from divulging: that you can hit almost any note and it won't sound too bad. Furthermore, if you hold down relentlessly on the "sustain" pedal, on the far right, the notes tend to blend into some kind of noise. The truth is simply to hear it with, as they say, your own internal ear and hope you do not awaken anyone who might say, like my daughter about the milk, "how disgusting!"

There is nothing I can recommend to the frayed physician better than a dash of "music," a wee Sonatina before retiring. At these times, however, you must also remember to press relentlessly down on the far left pedal to soften the sound. (Nobody, by the way, has ever figured out what the middle pedal is for, some saying simple "decor" and others seeing in it a religious symbolism, a "trinity" of pedals so to speak.) In any case, that I should even pretend to be attempting to play the piano, with any pedal at all, at my delicate age, astonishes me, and leaves me hopeful that anything, after all, may be possible in the universe.

Part of my astonishment lies in my discovery that you can actually learn to "do" music almost like surgery or the computer, even if you have no ear whatsoever. There is, after all, a Pythagorean formula, a rational method in the madness of it all that gradually becomes perceptible in spite of oneself. Anyway, I take comfort in Gustav Holst's wise and liberal words, thinking I understand precisely his meaning, that "if a thing is worth doing at all, it is

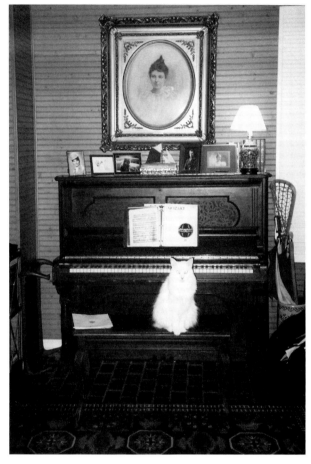

My grandmother and her piano, a rosewood and ivory Steinway upright,
given to her in 1896 before her marriage. She died in 1906, at age 33.

worth doing badly." Whether or not, in this litigious time, the premise applies to the practice of medicine, I leave you to decide.

The "Universal Truth" is accordingly that across a certain spectrum of life's opportunity, Holst's happy perception . . . namely, that you do not have to be the best or even particularly good in order to enjoy this or that . . . is worth taking comfort from. For years I was enslaved to the great Universal UnTruth, taught me ever since I was weeded out of a 150-voice choir in the 2nd grade and cast forth from the world of music into shame, that I was hopeless at any form of music whatsoever. No one in my family played a musical instrument any more than they flew a P-40 or a jet fighter. And yet there, sadly and silently shaming us all, still functioning and in good tune, was my grandmother Nellie's old upright Steinway, given to her in 1896 at the time of her marriage. If not Grand, it is a lovely old instrument, the keys real ivory, yellowed as we were told in my youth by her tuberculosis. Except for nasty forays against it when my sister and I would try to bang out a Chopsticks variation, it had been silent since her death in 1906.

A mixture of guilt and desire, great movers of the world, finally overcame the reluctance I had taught myself in order (Ezra Pound, I think) "that a Blunt should open." Accordingly, eight or nine years ago I started fooling with Nellie's lovely piano, using the "very quiet" pedal by night. I have fooled along, albeit I have not yet, any more than Dracula, come out to play by day; but I now see that anything is possible.

As a matter of fact, by the time you read this I will be "out of the closet." Soon I intend to start playing even by day. I am even filled with hope that my family will contrive to say things more nearly like "how beautiful!" rather than "how disgusting!" Who knows?

In any case, I am glad herewith to offer a real bit of thanks to the emergency room for having brought me to this point where I think I can almost play the piano a little bit. Bravely, after all, I have gone where none since my grandmother has ever gone before.

And if worse comes to worst, and I am pronounced still musically "disgusting," I can yet take comfort in "Jet Fighter II," with "III" in the offing.

Or, come to think of it, take up the bagpipe by night, loudly even, for much is possible, despite what we are taught.

SPEAKS STILL THE PAST

On the wall of my "exam room" hangs a wicked looking knife. It is draped horizontally over two nails and is a somewhat unattractive presence. It is surrounded by the usual pictures and diplomas, including the "kindergarten diploma" given me by the nice nurses when I finished my residency in plastic surgery at Shands Teaching Hospital.

This sinister blade has come, however, to overshadow all the other charming bits of memorabilia that surround it, including the wonderful picture of my mother, looking like a Joan Crawford stand-in, which appeared in a 1941 issue of *Town and Country*. It even eclipses the gorgeous picture of a beautiful young lady in her wedding gown, age 24, taken within a few months of a mastectomy and reconstruction sufficient to the moment's need. Beyond any presence on that wall, new patients commented on her beauty, happily complimented by the new husband at her side who looks like a cross between Mel Gibson and Tom Cruise.

Now everyone immediately fixates on this ugly knife, broad of blade, curving in right menacing fashion, its connotations somehow made all the worse by having a bright orange, pseudo-plastic handle.

Although my patients, particularly the new ones, hopeful and expecting God knows what, are taken a bit aback by this austere symbol, I am determined to let it be, for sweet sentiment's sake.

I have, however, had to develop a formula in reply to their question, slightly wan, "Is that what you use to do your surgery with, ha-ha?"

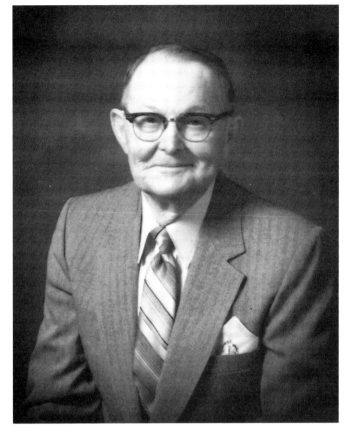

Mr. Tom Trawick.

"Ha-ha," I say, with a merry twinkle in my eye. "For the most part, no," and so on, with further words calculated by my intuitive interpretation of the patient's resiliency and sense of the absurd.

I go on, after completing these light bits of jocund banter, to explain the veritable facts, namely, that I had for many years an old gentleman patient who, afflicted by basal and squamous cell carcinomas of the face and neck, had tenderly undergone my scalpel from time to time, including a radical neck dissection and a few flaps turned from here and there. What an honorable, what a marvelous patient he had been! He was one of those individuals, allowing now a certain passion into my voice, who was a window into a time a century ago. A Georgia countryman, he was one of those sorts who had almost never been outside his own county. He had been born and bred to his church, born and bred to a pioneer work ethic and that natural graciousness and humor which our own world can only wish it possessed more of. Twice a year he would bring us not just one but two marvelous country hams, prepared by his own hand and, of course, with the knife that he had used for so many years.

A happy little bond grew between us, for such is the physician's privilege, and I would meet him from time to time at a pit barbecue restaurant half way between up there in Georgia and down here in Tallahassee, for barbecue and turnip greens, sweetened iced tea and other trimmings, to reminisce about mules and hard times in the depression. When he died, I felt him to be the last, or almost the last, of a frontier species which will soon be extinct and which we can legitimately mourn.

But wait! Not quite yet are they all gone, for I have just lunched with another gentleman of almost identical vintage albeit from a more privileged vineyard, who happily lives on in our midst. It was a different menu and venue, for this was a gentleman-physician honored by all in Tallahassee, and indeed throughout the state, Dr. George Palmer. And why not write, even if he is yet alive, a pleasant word of Dr. Palmer, and at that specifically in juxtaposition with old Tom Trawick, above noted. Yes, "let us now praise famous men," while they are yet capable of enjoying that bit of affection we can extend them. After all, here is a southern "gentleman of the old school," beloved by his patients and their parents during the many years since 1948 when he first opened his practice of pediatrics in Tallahassee. Gracefully wearing the mantle of numerous honors and appointments, it is worth remembering, particularly at this difficult time in the story of medicine in Florida, his comment on assuming the Presidency of the Florida Medical Association in 1966: "As long as we adhere to our principles and do what we think is right in our own hearts for the Association, for our patients, and

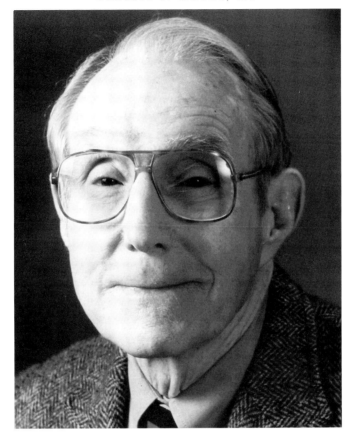

George S. Palmer, MD.

for the people we represent, we can hold our heads high, look anyone in the eye, and apologize to no one."

We lunched, not on this occasion upon barbecue but in elegant surroundings, although the food was no better. I soaked up the ambiance of Dr. Palmer. He speaks in easy tones with the accents of the cultured south, his voice modulated between an inherent gentility and the practiced softness of so many years soothing his patients, or rather his patients' moms and dads. He has the look of a septuagenarian Ashley Wilkes of Twelve Oaks Plantation. But if the manner is not dissimilar, the eyes are altogether different, for George Palmer's sparkle with good memories and the success of a life lived as a "good physician" should.

As I drove him home, after our luncheon in that lovely room full of lawyers, bureaucrats, legislators, and general potentates, he remarked at every corner on what once was. It is hard to believe so much has changed in a lifetime. Here was the little fruit stand on the corner run by old . . . whatever the name, forgive me . . . and here exactly behind the Capitol, standing on a brick street, had been his family home, now replaced by the Supreme Court building. Everything that was so small, so dusty, so well worn, so familiar to him as a boy is now paved and prepossessing.

But the honest human values of what was once upon a time a little southern town remain to him as if time had no meaning whatsoever.

They were values equally lived by my patient Tom Trawick. It seems to me that Dr. Palmer and Tom possess an affinity in their ways and means, so different in their circumstance yet so similar in their living it, that speaks to us still. Both kept their faith in the lives they led, whether as physician or patient.

Their way may be the best one can do in this universe. It is almost, even, a way of getting even with our ignorance.

Living or dead, they are worth our not forgetting.

[BRAVEHEART AMONGST US]

Allow me to introduce the following: The near-genuine article (edited alas!) written by one Colin Jamieson, now doctor of medicine, University of Manchester, England, 1996.

His professors, of course, forced him to write this essay on the pain of not receiving his degree, another of those impositions professors dream up before they allow young people to become entitled to all the perquisites and prerogatives of a doctorate in medicine.

You have read of Colin earlier. As you remember, I was astonished when his cousin, who dwells in Tallahassee, approached me to say that young Colin—at the time entering his fourth year of medical school—had to spend six weeks "somewhere else" in the world, to get some "perspective" on how medicine was practiced in elsewhere-wherever. Colin, "impecunious in serious fashion," was unable to afford the South of France, Italy, Hawaii, or Hong Kong and so took up his cousin's offer to spend six hot weeks here in little old Tallahassee, where he would have a roof over his head and a swimming pool, with my humble self as his medical chaperon.

Neither I nor anyone else in my office knew quite how we should behave. I pictured the arrival of a dour Scotsman, shaggy, with a great stick, a sheep tucked under one arm, a pipe clutched in his teeth, a haggis draped about his neck, and somewhere dimly stretching off to the horizon, a moor.

How to prepare for this apparition was the question. Our sainted office manager, Linda, bought some fresh plants for the office so he would not think we merely cultivate dead ones, and we purchased a tea pot.

Finally, dreadfully, the great day came, and Colin arrived.

Everyone immediately fell in love with him. He came equipped with a clear and open countenance, and so brilliantly rolled his r's that strong men felt weak and ladies swooned. We ourselves were smitten and immediately tried to get him to marry our oldest daughter (even though she was up in South Carolina) or, for that matter, to hang around and wait for the youngest. In other words, we threw ourselves at him for all we were worth. With great tact he fended off our every overture.

Thus was Colin exposed to the practice of American medicine. When he flew back to the University of Manchester and Scotland, he was forced to write about his experience here, to demonstrate he had actually gone somewhere, and so produced the following, which he was kind enough to send me. Let G.B. and H. herewith share this tidbit not only in honor of Colin, but as a worthwhile perspective on the American practice of medicine by an intelligent, charming young man.

ELECTIVE REPORT: LETTER FROM AMERICA

My journey began in Manchester. I had received a letter from one Dr. Moore, a plastic surgeon in Florida. The tone of the letter was polite and kind, but guarded, as if in answer to a rather unexpected question. This wary reply assured me of a place in the "Sunshine State" for a period of seven weeks with one condition: that I should endeavour to find a certain well-known book by the father of my chosen elective subject (plastic surgery).

Here, then, I found myself in the "wee sma hours" probing the deepest beer-can, shag-pile corners of the university in search of this glorious text. When all else had failed, I slipped a fiver to the librarian who smugly produced it that afternoon. "It's the only copy in all of Manchester, you know."

The book to which I am referring, of course, is The Principles and Art of Plastic Surgery by Sir Harold Gillies and Dr. Ralph Millard, the first, an inno-

vator of plastic surgical technique in World War I and the latter the famous American plastic surgeon who trained with Gillies in the 1950s.

So much has been written on this text that my contribution will have little effect on those who are aware of it. It is truly a remarkable book. As a medical student, one becomes inured to the boredom of navigating through mountains of "classic" textbooks, so it was a great surprise to read a book of what appeared to be anecdotes rather than stern instructions on the care of decubitus ulcers. I was struck that the people in the pictures had actually contributed their stories, expressing their feelings in a very personal way. Mr. Smith tells us a joke about his injuries received while shot down over France in World War I. Mrs. Brown, whose epilepsy caused her to fall face down in the fire, survives and makes some kind of life for herself.

As for Sir Harold and Dr. Millard, their commentaries on the development of plastic surgical techniques are interspersed everywhere with wit and humor, even at the darkest of times for their patients.

Dr. Moore's suggestion that I should glance at this book made me wonder more about him and what I would meet when I arrived.

My jet lag was relieved by a weekend in my cousin's swimming pool; I had sufficiently recovered to take on the world of plastic surgery myself.

Dr. Moore's practice surprised me.

As a Scotsman, I had been brought up in the Presbyterian Church of Scotland by stern practitioners who are recognized worldwide for their moral perseverance, irresistible grace, and some might say "dourness."

In this setting, plastic surgery has received bad press: the preserve of the rich, vulgar and, worst of all, the vain. My countrymen are entitled only to that which has been God given. In essence, Scottish people stay "ugly."

Then, were Dr. Moore's patients all that abhorrent to my Scottish character? The answer is "no."

The people who passed through his office were decent ordinary folk who wouldn't have looked out of place queuing at the co-op on the west side of the Kilmarnock. What, then, was the difference? The first thing is cultural acceptance. It is no more "improper" to visit a plastic surgeon in the States than it would be to visit a dentist here. One of the greatest assets the Americans possess is an openness and welcoming to other's ideas and values. People who want to improve themselves in whatever way are encouraged and supported. In the words of my friend Dr. Moore, the place of cosmetic surgery is to "help people become more like themselves"—a rather lovely phrase to my mind.

The other difference, I think, is also cultural in that vanity, money, possessions, etc., are acceptable and highly valued in American society.

Everyone in America is related to a Scot when they remember where Scotland is (just mention Highlander, Braveheart, or Rob Roy, and watch their misty eyes!).

This may be a testament to the Scottish wanderlust or, more insidiously, the virility of the Scots. In any event, Scottishness was a great introduction to the many characters I met on my travels. I enjoyed a couple of weeks observing Dr. Moore in action—rhinoplasties, abdominoplasties, and a whole host of lumps, bumps, spider nevi, and moles, moles, and more moles. Tallahassee is medically famous for two things: allergies and moles!

To watch Dr. Moore work was a pleasure. Much of this good work was done with the effects of Ketamine, a drug Dr. Moore swears by. A "side effect" of Ketamine allowed conversation with the on-table patients to their enlightenment as to the Scotsman's taste for haggis. I am guilty, I fear, of promoting the popular myth of the "haggis" and am unsure if I have left an indelible mark on these patient's subconscious. Needless to say "Haggi" are now roaming free in the orange groves of North Florida, perhaps providing the occasional lunch for a hungry alligator!

As part of my experience, I was sent to Atlanta, home of the High Museum, Emory University, and Scarlett O'Hara. I didn't see her, but I don't give a damn.

I was on a more serious mission to observe the amazing Dr. Carl Hartrampf perform his world-famous Transverse Abdominal Island Hartrampf flap (a fact that will only impress plastic surgeons).[1]

Dr. Hartrampf is only what can be described as wizardly. In his operating room I was entertained all day by great shouts of "yippee!" and "hurrah!" as a blood supply was expressed or a flap neatly tucked. The theatre nurses wrote jokes on sterile cards for all to see, rather than hear, as Dr. Hartrampf is gently tending towards presbycupia. In a corner, behind the anesthetist machine, that lady donned a false nose, spectacles and mustache, one by one the surgeons noticing her, and one by one dismissing her existence without comment. As a final accolade Dr. Hartrampf invited me to sign the "Hartrampf Visitor's Book."

All of the above is certifiably true.

In addition to plastic surgery, I spent time with various doctors at Tallahassee Memorial Hospital. My thanks go to Eric Norton, Charles Williams, Curt Kraft, Terry McCoy, Jack MacDonald, and Jim Totten. With these doctors I received a taste of family practice, radiology, and anesthetics.

From my experience in these specialities, it became clear to me just how much American medical practice is driven by money and litigation.

The Americans have persuaded themselves that if they become unwell it is somebody's fault, and if they are not 100 percent cured it is the doctors' fault, and if they die somebody must pay. The cycle goes on and on, helping no one. Doctors must practice "defensive medicine," patients pay huge insurance and pharmacy costs, and litigation takes up a large portion of hospital budgets and time. The figures are truly incredible.

---

[1] Dr. Hartrampf was the first to conceive and perform this flap, by which breast reconstruction is elegantly accomplished through moving skin and fat from the lower abdomen up onto the chest. The lady gains back her lost breast, and loses her unwanted "tummy." Dr. Hartrampf himself, as Dr. Jamieson notes, is to plastic surgery in Atlanta what Margaret Mitchell was to literature.

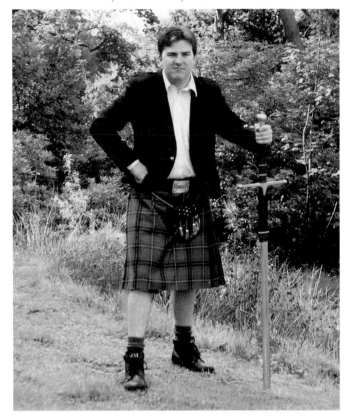

Braveheart and the Sword of Wallace.

I pray that with the current changes in the NHS we will not completely embrace the American dream. I am led to feel, in conclusion, that our own system, for all of its faults, possesses a rational approach to the practice of medicine, and a humane one too, which I fear may be seriously threatened in the American model. Theirs is an example of the mess that comes from attempting to mix big government, big business, and medicine.

My journey came to a close. What an experience!

I pondered what to do next.

FACTS ARE FACTS, BUT ART IS A MESS

The trouble with art, and come to think of it, with love, faith, hope, charity, and the practice of medicine, is that these do not readily translate into computer-speak. In the world of big government, big business, and big HMOs, art—and the previously noted virtues—is accordingly incapable of inclusion into those great computational equations and algorithms that now are used to define the tolerable practice of medicine. As Joe Friday was wont to say, "just the facts, Ma'am." In our case, the "facts" often have more to do with caring for the criteria than for the patient. Patience, a gentle touch, and a kind word may be lost as parameters of care.

To put it otherwise, more and more we must practice medicine by the numbers. These, we know, will be scrutinized by those who have become the accountants of our profession, and scrutinized with all the obsessiveness for which accountants are deservedly acclaimed. The numbers are, however, everywhere, not to forget that most important one which places a "$" sign in front of it.

Thus I was thinking the other day while I was working away, I think, at some wart. Pausing in my progress, I gazed raptly out the more or less clerestory windows of the room the patient and I were in, and saw clouds and leaves. Such a wonderful balance of order and chaos in nature, thought I, of number and numberlessness. "How do you count what a cloud is made of?" I queried the patient, my knife poised above the wretched wart. I received no answer, or perhaps one so muffled as to be unintelligible.

"Never mind," I said. "You are doing very well, and the wart has met its doom." I gave her a little pat, as well as words of gentle assurance in my most considerate tone of voice.

No computer was there to mark our pleasant exchange. Such an exchange, after all, is made of the same stuff as clouds, wonderfully shaped, but hard to grasp, and impossible for a computer, which knows only CPT codes[1] and the paltry facts as to whether "wart removal" is or is not covered under the terms of the HMO contract.

With the happy patient merrily on her way, and having five or ten minutes to myself, I decided to grow a little petulant. Petulance, after all, is still allowed if reasonably kept to oneself.

Thus tempted, but still capable of saving myself, I popped next door where exist the chambers of that noble organization, The Capital Medical Society. Actually, it was Mollie Hill, the Executive Directrix of our society who I wanted to visit, along with her estimable sub-Directrix Rosalie. I thought it would cheer me up, as dark thoughts prevailed upon my brain, to look at Mollie's desk, or to discover if there was a tidbit of gossip she might share. Mollie, after all, knows everything there is to know about how medicine is practiced in Tallahassee—and pretty much how it is practiced elsewhere, too. She flies to Chicago and Miami to attend great meetings. She has heard Hillary Clinton speak. She assimilates all; she sees and hears with the nicest intelligence.

She is the veritable oil that bathes the mighty pistons of the medical machine which beats back disease in Tallahassee. It is doubtless that you have a person like her at your own society, but I am prejudiced to think that Mollie is *primus inter pares*, a veritable *capo di capi*. Her "quality" is in no need of "Assurance."

---

[1] A compilation which rigorously attempts to quantify diseases and treatments so that some computer, if it is working, will pay physicians, or not, depending on how the computer feels that day, for their services.

As I walked down the short hallway to her office, my petulance was arrested by the sight of sheets of letter-size paper, placed at strategic intervals on the floor, with arrows pointing toward her office door. Boldly written on each sheet were various phrases: "DANGER!" . . . "HORRORS AHEAD!" . . . "GO NO FURTHER!" . . . "DON'T FORGET, WE WARNED YOU!" Intrigued, I followed these threats—warnings—to the threshold of Mollie's office. I peeked in cautiously, then staggered back, my titanium hips and grubby knees turned to jello by the wonderful state of disarray—no, chaos—that reigned within. So covered was it with weighty documents that no floor was to be seen! Pile upon pile of random letters, articles, magazines, assorted nondescript paper, and pink "Call Me Back" messages littered her desk. It was a scene beyond any computer's ability to fathom.

In the midst of this mess sat Mollie, calmly computing. In the midst, veritably of apparent chaos, intelligent life flourished! "The brain," thought I, remembering Miss Dickinson's poem:

...is wider than the sky,
For, put them side by side,
The one the other will include
With ease, and you beside.

Mollie functions beyond the analytical parameters, and so do we physicians, too, I thought. I felt my petulance abating. I took hope, and saw before me as though I had dreamt the possibility, again, of physicians being raised above the petulant, constrictive criteria that are now used by committees to define quality of care and utilization of resources. My spirit soared toward the empyrean.

"Well, what brings you over here? We haven't seen you for awhile! Where have you been?" she asked, in a vaguely accusatory manner.

"I've been nowhere, of course, what do you expect? I'm just barely next door, as you may recall. Neither you nor Rosalie ever come to visit me, so

I thought I would quit visiting you until you visited me." I felt a little petulance rising in my spleen. "But I couldn't hold out," I added wimpily, even though with Mollie I knew you should never, ever appear "wimpish."

I think she sniffed at me slightly, and turned back to her computer screen. I asked her if she knew any gossip, which she, being busy, rejected as a valid question. So, I asked her about the state of medicine in Tallahassee and the nation. To this question, she was more responsive, because she thought that I just might, on the basis of her reply, contrive some article for our local newsletter. She will, somewhat cynically I think, do anything for "copy."

"You have all lost it. Doctors are out there signing contracts without even reading them.

"Accordingly, you will deserve all, or rather what little, you get," she said, I thought even more cynically.

"But how can anyone read them?" I asked. "I never do."

She sniffed again, as though to say, "I told you so, poor fool"—her sniff filled with disdain.

"Well, don't sniff at me," I retorted, "just look at this mess your office is in, poor Rosalie alarmed to the extent that she has had to put down warnings to all who enter at their own risk. The JCAH would never accredit you!"

"And I don't have to give a damn," she said. "Out of muddle I make meaning. And so should you."

I crouched at her feet while she lectured me on how women, and men, too, should stand up for themselves and take the raw material of chaos and mold it into beautiful form; that we should read our contracts and all that mess, but rise above them; and that by being shrewd about the facts we can also take the feelings, that chaos of feelings beyond any computer's power to weigh, and make again the practice of medicine an art that treats the whole patient and not merely computers or committees or HMOs or the government.

Again, my spirit soared. I felt uplifted to have visited such an oracle, seated as she was in the midst of a mess in front of a computer rather than on a tripod. "Would that it could be once more," I thought, skipping back to my office. "In the midst of this mess we now must practice within, all we have to do is to be good."

It may seem to you a *non sequitur*, but later that day, in response to a vague question by my 14-year-old daughter, I said to her, sagely I thought, "Never trust a man with a perfectly clean desktop, or perfect statistics."

"Oh," she said. But, I knew what I meant anyway.

IN THE REAL WORLD,
IMAGE IS MONEY

I do not want to hear from all you hard-working family practitioners, internists, gall bladder surgeons, and bone-setters that doing plastic surgery is some sort of mere lighthearted frivolity.

There is no telling, of course, what Benjamin Franklin might have said about it. But if in his day he said, "Time is money," I think nowadays he might have rephrased the remark to "Image is money."

Take a look at Madonna. Her image earns her more in 10 seconds than we pitiful time-servers will earn in a lifetime.

A big image pays big bucks, and you don't even have to worry about whether your image is good or bad, although the latter seems to fetch more than the former.

Image, even in the animal world, is a big step toward success. Oh, true, those hard-working sheep dogs in Scotland get a nod of public approval, working as they do in all kinds of weather—through rain and snow and fog—for not much more than a bowl of hot oatmeal at the end of a hard day. It is Lassie and Rin-Tin-Tin who made the big money, because they had the image thing all worked out. We are beguiled by Lassie's tail feathers, her noble ruff, and her elegant length of nose.

The nose, of course, has a great deal to do with image. Madonna's nose is fairly striking I think; Barbra Streisand's is inviolable as an icon; and, of course, who could possibly conceive of Charles de Gaulle with a dinky nose?

I was prompted to these thoughts the other day while I was idly leafing through *Horse Illustrated*, a journal I avoid like the plague because we have a horse, and the very thought of horse makes my checkbook sweat and tremble. My eye, however, was caught by an article titled "Equine Rhinoplasty." Eagerly I read the report, thrilled that a whole new population of horses might need nose jobs. Like lawyers, we have too many plastic surgeons, and so need more noses, just as they need more litigation.

In any case, I was intrigued to see that poor Double Diamond Sue had been chased into a fence by some horses and broke her nose. A huge lump was left on her nasal dorsum, and the awful fact loomed that her show career might be over. Double Diamond Sue, according to the article, was in luck, for she was referred to a real, live, board-certified plastic and reconstructive surgeon, Dr. John Emery. Emery did an examination and, like the ancient Egyptian physicians would say, pronounced, "This is a case I will take."

Dr. Emery, the article went on, astutely noted that nose jobs on horses were different from those performed on humans, observing that the horse's nose is a lot bigger. Double Diamond Sue was not anesthetized, but simply sedated, and in the highest tradition of the horse, stood through the entire operation—without even the benefit of a twitch. This is an anesthetic method that involves putting a massive clothes-pin-like clamp on the horse's lower lip, and twisting it sufficiently so the horse is totally preoccupied by what is going on with its lip. Major surgery can be performed, and if movement occurs, the horse anesthetist tightens the clamp.

I do not know if Dr. Emery has attempted this method on human patients, but I congratulate him, because Sue's image was fully restored, and she is now back on the money-making circuit.

Double Diamond Sue's story demonstrates the secure place that plastic surgery now enjoys within the armamentarium of means we use to get through life. After all, we are always trying to make ourselves better or to keep what we once had. It is an image thing that goes deep. To stay reasonably attractive has meaning in this highly competitive modern world where youth, and not looking grotesque, is placed at such value. (Not to deny youth the pleasures of over-sized shorts with the waist somewhere around the pubis.)

It is nothing to laugh about. Try presenting yourself to a potential employer with an unrepaired cleft lip in the hope of getting a job dealing with the public; or go to a cocktail party without your nose. Deformities in our world must be kept as hidden, except on the front page of the *National Enquirer*, as F.D.R. once had to hide his wheelchair, and even subtle aberrations catch our eye.

At least we do not practice death by exposure of children anomalously afflicted, and the cleft lip is no longer a mark of the devil, points that allow me the hope that mankind advances in its sensitivity.

We are all seeking "image enhancement," and the financial remuneration that we hope stems therefrom. We even pay to go to seminars to find out how to appear to look better than we are. One of the great successes of the Internet is that people can make themselves up, presenting themselves as they wish, for example: six feet, two inches tall, athletic, and loving to walk in the rain, or five feet, six inches tall, playful, and enjoying quiet dinners.

Poor Double Diamond Sue! She lives in the real world where a bump on the nose is intolerable. A good horse simply must look her best at all times. Image, though philosophers may deny it, is a "quality of life" point in our world.

I must get a couple of mirrors and look at my nose in profile. Even though the image-debilitating zit I had on it a couple of months ago is gone, I wonder if Dr. Emery could do something for me? But not standing up, please!

Hoofnote: Not wanting to prejudice my thoughts with facts, this essay was written before I called Dr. Emery, a charming gentleman-surgeon out in San Francisco. I told him how much he had stimulated my own hopes to find a horse on which I could do a nose job. He said that the surgery was easy as falling out of a saddle, the horse being given only a little Rompon, a dissociative agent, and some Xylocaine. In a dream state the horse just stands there and permits you to do your worst. No twitch was used; but it is the upper lip that is twitched, not the lower, in case you want to try this technique on any of your friends or, perhaps, an attorney.

THE SCAN IS QUICKER BUT ART IS THICKER

I consider myself, if forced to admit it, an Oslerian (Sir William, that is) minus the scholarship, the patience, the perceptive eye, the degrees and honors, the *humanitas*, the *gravitas*, and of course the mustache. One can naturally, even so, always hope, which is surely one of the values of "heroes" in their stimulation of us towards themselves. I suppose I could conceivably grow a mustache, of sorts, but scarcely Oslerian in its *veritas* since I lack a sufficiently fertile upper lip. Indeed, I could almost better aspire to the prospect of being made Regius Professor of Medicine, ODE, DPhil, etc., at Oxford or winning 10 million dollars in the Publisher's Clearinghouse Sweepstakes.

But let me not limit, God forbid herein, our and even my own human potential! It does the very name "Osler" injustice, and must not be.

And yet even he had to reconcile himself to certain limitations, even if blandness of the upper lip was not one of them. He had, after all, to engage in the study and practice of medicine lacking almost the least Technology which we so merrily take for granted. He was forced to practice medicine purely as an Art, an art which some might say he personifies as having brought to its finest acme. Of course, the rapidly developing knowledge of Science as it applied to medical practice he readily, indeed eagerly, incorporated into his art, but as for technology it was almost nonexistent as we now know it in his years. One hundred years later art remains of course (it always must), but Technology, massive and a little monstrous, has displaced it on the altar we worship before. Nor do I mean to treat technology in a pejorative

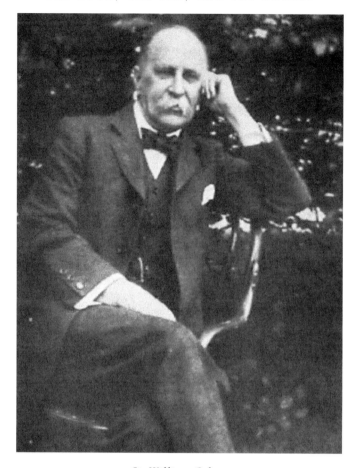

Sir William Osler.

sense; for there is nothing more marvelous than the CAT scan, or the happy removal on even an outpatient basis of one's gallbladder by way of a shiny little tube. Art, indeed, pales somewhat before such accomplishment.

When it comes to our latter day "bottom line," however, Technology costs a lot more than Art. Even Osler would be as daunted as we in knowing how best to cut the deal between the cost-effectiveness of medicine practiced as an Art (looking at the patient's tongue, checking the pulse, holding the hand) and the cost-extravagance of practicing it as a Technology (CAT scans for every headache). He was a marvelous answer for his time, and still for ours as well, and embodies that happy image of the Doctor as Physician-Philosopher, the High Priest of Health, and the practitioner of medicine not only by virtuosity but as Virtue.

How, in our day, when ways and means seem to overshadow people and their places, does one live up to such ideals? I myself, practicing as an old-fashioned, country plastic surgeon, would beyond measure startle my patients and colleagues if suddenly I presented myself as "a High Priest of Health," and donned the robes of Virtue fully fledged. People would laugh, and even Osler would in all likelihood sadly shake his head. Osler lived in a world where lofty ideals were granted unquestioned respect, and we in one eroded by relativism, where "high" values appear presumptuous, almost suspect.

And yet we can still sneak them in, can't we? In the midst of all these lawyers, managed-care bureaucrats, and massive technological apparati there yet remains the singular physician who, in his or her relationship with a patient, defines the humanity of that contact. The art of doing so wisely and well is what will save us from being subject to the lawyers and our own Technology.

In art, by which I now mean pictures, music, and so on, the changes that occur in style and vision reflect the temper of the times, and so also does the art of medical practice become modified. As I read over Osler's *Aequanimitas*, as is titled his valedictory address to the graduating students of the University of Pennsylvania Medical School given in May 1889, I know that I cannot practice *aequanimitas* any more than I can do *gravitas*, or grow a great mustache. A bit foreign to me is the physician who possesses such divine "imperturbability . . . coolness and presence of mind under all circumstances, calmness amidst storm, clearness of judgment in moments of grave peril, immobility, impassiveness, or, to use an old and expressive word, *phlegm*." My patients, I fear, would be appalled and scattered by my attempts at "phlegm." For our egalitarian age, the Physician-on-Pedestal-Imperturbable does not quite do, at least here just south of the Georgia line. Osler departs from his Valedictory saying to us, "Gentlemen—Farewell, and take with you into the struggle the watchword of the good old Roman *Aequanimitas*."

It makes me want to whimper, quite in contrast to Osler's dictum in fact, marveling that in a mere one hundred years I could, as a medical practitioner, have been brought so low from the Oslerian ideal.

But wait! This speech of Osler's, this *aequanimitas*, was a Valedictory address, which necessarily doomed his words to a high flight of serious purpose. The man himself, for all the mustache, had another side, which must not be forgotten. In *Garrison's History of Medicine*, Dr. Arnold Klebs notes Osler's personality as a teacher, "Urging, encouraging, inspiring, so we saw him always exact, dogmatic never, and when the humorous friendly fire kindled in his eyes you could not help but love him, and with him the task we had chosen for our life work." For all the *Gravitas et Aequanimitas* there is, for sure, a rich *Humanitas*. The success Osler so wonderfully achieved in almost inventing the teaching of clinical medicine in America must be credited not merely to his indefatigable enthusiasm for the work at hand, but his good humor as well, which made friends of both colleagues and, I would guess, patients too.

No, I am not sure how much *Aequanimitas* we need incorporate in our practices these days, other than perhaps for the pathologists, some neurosurgeons, and an occasional dermatologist attempting to manage an itch; and even they, among the rest of us, if we are to save ourselves from managed care and pure technocracy, will do so as a result of the good humor, the interest, and the kind moment we can give to a worried patient, hurting and afraid. Nothing will beat that.

You don't need a great mustache for it. You don't need to be swathed in the robes of Regius Professor for it. You don't need to have done a hundred postmortems, or have studied with, or even read, Koch. We can yet in our post-modern way live up to the Oslerian tradition, even if it is hard to pronounce *Aequanimitas*.

On which hopeful note, and because the chance might be slightly higher than that of my becoming Regius Professor of Medicine at Oxford, I must now go mail at my daughter's insistence the form she has filled out, and which she is certain we will win, making us contestants in the Publisher's Clearinghouse Sweepstakes. She asked me, if she wins the 10 million dollars for us, what car I would buy? A Lexus?

"No," I said, "I think I'll get something with a little more *Humanitas*." I thought a moment, and then said artfully, "Maybe I'll even keep my old 1979 Toyota."

THE
BAD

INTRODUCTORY: THE BAD

In this, the Great Age of Relativism, a dominant feature of the Zeitgeist of our times is that things are good or bad only insofar as we perceive them to be in relation to whatever else. We forgive ourselves and everyone else much as a result, which is no bad thing either. As a plastic surgeon I am grateful every day for the generosity of my patients who are content enough with improvements relative to their former circumstance, and let it go at that. And yet, of course, there might be in the offing a truly "Bad" result, for example (I can scarcely write it) sudden death on the operating room table; or even permanent damage to a facial nerve branch during the course of a "facelift," or myriad lesser matters that fall short of the "Good" one is wishing to achieve.

No matter what say the Relativists, nor no matter how tepid the mix of hot and cold within which we live, Bad is perhaps more easily identified than Good, and when it happens to ourselves its mitigating circumstances sound pretty hollow in the ear. When Bad is really bad, even the most confirmed relativist grows a little quiet, I do believe.

At some point, finally, Bad cannot be forgiven by anyone. In the spring of 1998, I took our now 15-year-old daughter and a girl friend of hers to Amsterdam, in large measure conceiving the trip as a pilgrimage most appropriate to the moment of my daughter's years, and my own as a Dad. There is, after all, no publicly accessible place, to my knowledge, where that dichotomy between Good and Evil is so sharply brought to focus as those tiny rooms where Anne Frank lived her last years. And then, that she should be so brutally torn from that narrowest confinement, the papers of her diary left indiscriminately scattered on the floor, and be taken to worse horrors and death, strikes one like a burst of Darkness far off the scale of "relative values."

Happily I have, as I would guess have also most of the people who might read these essays, lived in a moderate and even privileged world, spared much. Those immemorial siblings, death and disease, dwell further from us than once they did; divorce is our most public pain, nor need we deny the simple, wearisome accumulation of sundry day-to-day vicissitudes such as flat tires, a flat breast (if the implant was saline filled), a computer breakdown, and the inability to get a real, live, human person on the other end of the phone line. These are paltry matters, and homely too, but yet add their small weight into the balance.

Thus you will find these minor concerns of my own, listed so presumptuously as "Bad." Most are not particularly bad at all. I tend to rant on about bureaucracy and HMOs, suspecting them . . . while at the same time recognizing their need and value too . . . as being liable to succumb to the solipsisms implicit in their existence, which ultimately may become more for the sake of themselves than the people they are meant to serve. Am I wrong, or did not Hitler himself, separated from the death camps by reams and realms of bureaucrats, forbid the mentioning in his presence of what all knew?

Nor are you to think that because there is a spate of articles about "The Breast" included in this section that I think, as an organ, the breast is "bad." Far from it, I assure you. In its honor, indeed, I have written a separate introductory essay to this topic, for in truth I am as enamored of the breast, and the lovely curves of its ideal shape, as much as any man, if not a little more, for I have had the privilege of being permitted its close study as an aesthetic shape. The Bad here has nothing to do with the breast, but all to do with its plunder by the media and, more lately, the judiciary establishment. That the media, by way of our televisions, could march into the family rooms of perfectly healthy and happy ladies in possession of a bit of silicone, and by carefully orchestrated words and images terrify them, was unconscionable. That the lawyers cheered the media on, their path cleared by self-righteous activists in their pay, on evidence so flimsy as to be scientifically and rationally negligible, was nothing but egregious self-serving. It may now be the "American Way," but the fact that billions of dollars later, and numerous entire bits of the nation's industry destroyed, and the emotional well-being of two million ladies thus preyed upon, seems to me, given the absence of evidence, "Bad" indeed.

Ah well, we shrug it off now. Those ladies, though scarred more of brain than bosom, have pretty much recovered. The country carries on. The breast (or two) remains on the cover of *Cosmopolitan*. We do not have to know those few lawyers who merrily divided up the billions, which is after all so huge a number as to be almost an abstraction.

Such mismanagements, bad though they may be for a couple of million people and a tiny handful of plastic surgeons who were suddenly forced into the practice of psychiatry, are easily enough assimilated. So are the other bits of "Bad" I chose to think as such, and pondered ever so slightly upon. I admit that I have been blessed . . . never having been either (seriously) sued or audited by the IRS . . . and have been happily spared that embittering anguish that so many have so unfairly had thrust upon them.

I live, in fact, a life of rather tepid circumstance, where little goods and little bads flirt and flow about each other, where cold and hot mingle, and I am neither scalded nor frozen when I enjoy the benison of my bath. It is a most moderate life, with which I am most humbly and yet immoderately content. Even "Bad," as you shall see, is pretty good.

EVEN IN VERMONT...

I am being *slightly reflective. For the sake of the mood, I have cast about my shoulders a cloak of inky black. I have fashioned about my head not a cloud of dust like Pigpen's in* Peanuts, *but a grey mist suitable for elegies in country church yards. I sit at an antique secretary-*desk, a real pen in hand. As I glance through the wavy panes of the mullioned windows at my right, I see, indeed, a lovely church immediately across the street, complete with ancient gravestones rising out of the ground like ghosts.

It is snowing. The falling snow mutes all sounds from without. The world is ahush, and except for the crackling fire to my left the only sounds I hear are in my head, like scampering mice or the ding dongs of half-forgotten memories suddenly aroused.

As I sit here, poised between past and future in the Old Tavern at Grafton, Vermont, in the veritable room where Rudyard Kipling once sat in those awkward days of his venture to America, I think, prosaically enough, that "time flies." I know of no thought so commonplace, and yet so preternaturally and invariably shocking. It has been a hundred years since Kipling sat here; but that to me is an abstraction. It has been 25 years ago since I was here, which seems dumbfounding.

But let's get down the facts! In these past 25 seasons of falling snow since I was a general surgery resident at the Mary Hitchcock Hospital in Hanover, New Hampshire, a few miles up the road from Grafton, I mildly reflect on the great changes that have occurred in medicine in that interim. First are the technological advances, by which somehow I mostly mean CT scans and the ability to take gall bladders out through a small tube; "managed care," a concept almost beyond comprehension 25 years ago; and ultimately the rise of the lawyer as medical practitioner and arbiter of that care.

Given Kipling's own experience in this very place, it is this latter point I ponder. He himself, just down the road from Grafton, was served a bitter dose of the American character at its litigious best. As I thought of his experience, I pondered, weak and weary, on how well nigh minuscule was my own awareness of legal intimidation as it applied to the practice of medicine 25 or 30 years ago. I almost think that the very first time it ever dawned on me, practically, that doctors could be sued, was at the Mary Hitchcock. During my four-year surgery residency at that institution, there were two cases that caused rumbling of which I was a bit aware.

One related to a burn patient. The burn was severe, something like 75 percent of the total body surface area. The treatments included Neosporin ophthalmic ointment to the eyes. The patient, good grief, developed a panophthalmitis, and went blind. His life was saved, but the cause of the blindness was ultimately discovered to be contamination, if you can believe it, of the Neosporin ointment with some sort of resistant bacterium. I think there was a suit, which either came to nothing or perhaps was settled; I have no idea for sure. But I was impressed, and left shaking in my scrubs, the lesson being that even the most minor "applications" can have horrendous outcomes.

The other case involved me only peripherally, but scared us all. A young man, 17 or 18, underwent what I think was a pretty routine appendectomy, but bled in the aftermath. He kept on bleeding . . . and bleeding . . . and some 150 units later was transferred to Massachusetts General Hospital in Boston. Bleeding does not necessarily respect the reputation of an institution, and after a few more days and many more pints of blood he died even with the aid of the most sophisticated techniques. I heard rumors of litigation bruited about; but what it came to I never knew, for I was long gone before the stately progress of the law would have come to terms with that episode. One would go mad in the practice of medicine if one had to constantly expect the unexpected; but it is always there, lurking.

As for Rudyard Kipling, I do not know if he recorded at any point his own feelings about being sued in New England. They must have been bitter to an extreme. One does not picture Vermont as a suit-happy state; and if so little in 1968, how much less so in 1896 when Kipling was put through three years of misery and, finally, driven from our country as a result.

Kipling's wife, née Balestier of Dummerston, Vermont, had brought her husband, in the first flush of his fame, home to Vermont. Kipling had been smitten with the snow-bound landscape: "It was beautiful beyond expression, nature's boldest sketch in black and white, done with the Japanese disregard of perspective, and daringly altered from time to time by the restless pencils of the moon."

With plenty of money from his pen, and plenty of pretensions on the part of Mrs. Kipling, a grand house was built, on ten acres of land, land in part owned by her boisterous, ne'er-do-well brother. He gave them a portion of the property with the proviso that he should have the "mowing rights." On a part of this field, Mrs. Kipling created a formal garden, which became the *casus belli* between Kipling and his wife's brother. Insults were hurled at Kipling by his brother-in-law. Kipling himself was heard to say at an inn one day that, "Beatty is his own worst enemy. I have been obliged to carry him for the last year, to hold him up by the seat of his britches."

Beatty Balestier attempted to ride Kipling down with his horses as Kipling was out bicycling. "You've got to retract the God-damn lies you've been talking about me," shouted Beatty, "you've got to retract them in a week or by Christ I'll punch the God-damn soul out of you!" he shouted.

Kipling found himself suddenly in the toils of American law, succumbing the following week to the temptation to impose upon Beatty a warrant charging him with "assault with indecent and opprobrious names, and epithets, and threatening to kill."

The press loved it, of course. Kipling's privacy was utterly destroyed. A trial supervened with Kipling on the stand for two days, the lawyers probing him with the most intimate questions. The jury was in favor of their own boy, a native versus an alien, a Vermonter against the rich and famous Englishman.

The case went to a grand jury, but the publicity had been too much for Kipling. He dropped the charges, packed his belongings and his wife, and fled from Vermont forever. The large house was shut up.

Two and a half years later Kipling returned to America. The people of South Vermont now had high hopes that Kipling would return to them, and they could make amends. No such good fortune! In 1899, the press announced that Beatty Balestier was bringing an action against Kipling for $50,000 damages for "malicious persecution, false arrest, and defamation of character." The case was once again in the headlines. Kipling refused to return to Vermont, and the house was dismantled. Embittered, Kipling sailed for England, never to return to the United States.

And so, as the snow falls, I ponder life's irregularities, and the unpredictability of those "slings and arrows of outrageous fortune," which one can only hope to avoid. Even in Vermont, there is no escape, whether it be 1896 or 1996. In only six hours it will be 1997. I'm going to finish the year cautiously, and try not to slip in the shower as I dress for dinner. Over cocktails I am going to do my best not to hurl some vile epithet at anyone with a bushy mustache and thick glasses, who might be muttering something about Gunga Din. At dinner, I will chew my food carefully, so as to avoid as best I can having someone practice the Heimlich maneuver on me. Afterwards, I will stand by the fire, but not too close so as to cause my coat tails to combust. If I find myself in conversation with any attorneys, I am going to be particularly kind and gracious, and not step on their toes either accidentally or maliciously. I plan to tiptoe through these last hours of 1996 so that at midnight I may toast its passing as having been "good."

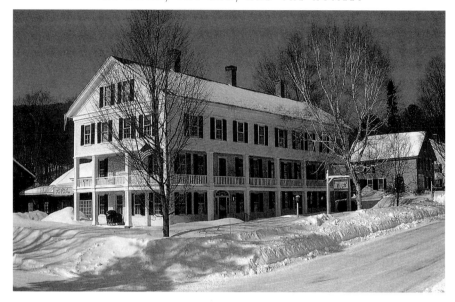

The Old Tavern, Grafton, Vermont.

Tomorrow, however, I am throwing caution to the wind! We are going cross-county skiing, me with my knee cartilages in shreds and my lovely titanium hips, suffused with a reckless New Year certainty that no "irregularities" will supervene.

Yet risk is anywhere, even in quiet New England. Just ask Kipling, who did a lot better on India's northwest frontier than in Vermont.

A HUMBLE,
HOMELY APOLOGY

Alas, *I feel compelled to confess to a homely, bad bit of rudeness I perpetrated on another physician this past month. I suppose such a lapse could be called quite* "unprofessional," *and the only exonerating circumstance I can come up with is that on the* whole I am, after all, the soul of courtesy.

It's all the fault, really, of Alexander Bell and his apparatus which, when it tinkles, our culture has trained us to think as an absolutely imperative summons, no matter what even highly private circumstance may be interrupted. In my case it was mere sweet sleep, I promise, but sleep thoroughly deserved, and physiologically much needed because I was trying to recover from an unfair virus which had settled in my nose, head, and perhaps spleen. I was also, of course, "on call" for that weekend and was, therefore, constrained from pulling the telephone wires from the wall. We do not have an answering machine, which could be turned off, because we have never much enjoyed coming home, say from the beach, and having to sit down immediately and go through a mess of messages that have accumulated.

Well, as I was saying, the Bell device has about its ringing an overbearing demand that we drop everything and fly to its insistence, trying to get there often at the risk of life and limb by the third or fourth ring. The response is almost Pavlovian, only you don't necessarily get a nice ham bone as a reward every time you respond to the bell. Still, it is all very dog-like, and perhaps you will allow me the pleasant fantasy of the days when messages were delivered bidding you respectively this or that, written in a pleasant copper plate, and left on a silver salver somewhere in the foyer. Of course, we do not have a copper plate or a silver salver, nor even a foyer. The front door at our house is a choking point, and when we have more than two couples over and they all try to leave at once we tend to jam up, getting arms and legs entangled, and only forcing the guests through the door with a final "pop." This spills them down the front stairs and with luck into their cars. It is not a graceful means of exit but it's the best we have been able to manage, and we refuse to move just for the sake of a commodious "entrance hall."

In any case, there is something to be said for writing a letter, even if the postage rates are going up yet again so that "nice" mail can pay for all the junk stuff. But I wander from my point, which had to do with the telephone tinkling at my bedside, circa 2:00 A.M., my nose stuffy, and my head full of phlegmon and fumes. I had a rather busy evening in the emergency room— a bit of a chainsaw in the face, a fingertip off, a windshield beveling down a forehead—and so was thoroughly deserving of a little decent rest and repose. As well, it was Friday night and I had yet two nights to be on call. I always feel if I can just squeak through Friday night without having to drag into the ER I can then negotiate Saturday and Sunday willy-nilly, and arrive at my office Monday morning at least a faint shadow of my Thursday's self. But if I am called in Friday night, I am then behind the 8-ball. If Saturday and Sunday are busy too, I become nothing but a ghostly wraith. Why is it that airline pilots, who sit in comfortable chairs doing almost nothing, get days and days off before they fly again; whereas we physicians are supposed to deal with real life and death matters and, no matter what, do it gracefully.

This "gracefully" business returns me to my graceless response to the phone call this recent Friday night.

It was, of course, the answering service cheerily directing me to call the emergency room of some small hospital that I had never dealt with way up in Georgia. I was given the number, and after fumbling in the dark with the buttons of my telephone, playing a variant of blindman's bluff and tic-tac-toe in the night, I ultimately reached this distant locale which I could only have desired to be a thousand miles or so even more distant at that moment. A doctor in the emergency room was finally placed on the phone, announcing briefly that some poor soul's ear had been torn off, and was "hanging by a thread." Now you have to start forgiving me: I can hardly bear that things are "hanging by a thread," because I picture a thread as being something with which one might sew on a button, at least a diameter of most tenuous dimension. Another problem, of course, with use of this sort of terminology, particularly with a doctor you are totally unfamiliar with, is that on occasion these "threads" really could be of much greater dimension, and even contain a complete vascular pedicle, maybe a nerve. But in this instance, aided and abetted by my stuffy nose and headache, I chose maliciously to accept the diagnosis that the ear was hanging "by a thread."

"Cut it off," I said, I fear quite gruffly but meaning then to go on to describe the usual protocol of chilling the part. I planned to de-epithelialize the cartilage, bury it in the remaining skin, and maybe in due course do a reconstruction. But I never got so far, the line apparently going dead. There was no sound of the telephone hanging up, just a sudden nothingness.

Thinking we had been cut off, I retrieved the telephone number once again from my answering service, having thoroughly forgotten it, and attempted to call the ER physician back. I was told that she refused to speak with me ever again, ever. I gathered that she was put out, and I felt much grieved by my own behavior. They are still quite furious with me up there, I know, and I spent the rest of my weekend feeling not only on call but morose with myself. It is all a bit bitter, and I am herewith offering apologies to the medical profession as a whole, and to that ER physician in particular, for my curmudgeonish attitude.

As for further moral conclusions from this episode, I herewith and henceforth resolve evermore to a more considered and placid response under such circumstances, begging myself to remember that it is "better to be called at 2:00 A.M. than never to be called at all."

On the other hand I don't think airline pilots have to fly for days, maybe even weeks, when and after they have a cold and runny nose. Another advantage they have, too, is that if they look out their window and notice a wing hanging "by a thread" there is not much point in worrying about it. As a matter of fact, the pilot might himself even say, "just cut it off."

ECONOMIC CREDENTIALING[1] AND THE HIGH COST OF KLEENEX

After careful consideration, duly aware that they have their problems too, I have come to the generous conclusion that I will not bill our local hospitals for $683,141.23. Maybe in return they will have the decency not to economically credential me.

I calculate this sum, by the way, to be the amount owed me for labors performed in behalf of these institutions over the past twenty years of true and honest service. Nor does this amount even take into account the immense quantity of good will and "free advertising" I have willingly dispensed in my own easy moments; for how many times, at some standing-around-party in reply to some other standing-around-party-goer who is about to be hospitalized, have I not lavished upon our hospitals encomiums of hearty praise?

"Yes, the nurses are so wonderful, and the food," I always say, "is superb. People come from miles around for the fried chicken." The understandably fearful patient leaves my presence comforted by my encouragements.

It is not for these positive remarks that I might attach, in the climate of our present moment, a crass monetary value. It is for the work done in the middle of the night on the Indigent Battered. Yet these patients come not so much to me but to the institution, which at any hour of the day or night I have been willing and proud to serve, never minding inconvenience, snow, or

[1]A perfidious, from the physician's point of view, plot on the part of hospitals to grant or remove a doctor's hospital privileges dependent on whether the physician turns a sufficient profit or (gasp!) lack of it for the hospital.

wildest storm (hurricane once, and all the lines were down, the trees tumbling about and chimneys falling).

No, not for me to cavil but to rush once more into that breech, upheld by the ideals of a long tradition. The ideal has been sufficient, for though I have never heard them say it, I have always chosen to feel that the hospitals I thus serve reciprocated both trust and support, even if I do admit a good number of Medicaid patients. I felt I was "stood behind" and that the hospital and I, supportive of each other's role, served happily the needs of our community and patients. That limb of The Triangle of Trust between doctor, patient, and hospital was (I thought) geometrically sound.

Well, times are bad and our professional ideals, which mean so much to us, are becoming mere commodities in the view of those forces that are so unscrupulously attempting to manipulate our fate.

Yes, even in Tallahassee, we have an unpleasant business going on. Not the mere specter, but the reality of "Economic Credentialing" is rampant in our midst! The hospital may cloak the issue in euphemism and the costly subtle jargon of its attorneys, but the facts seem eloquently clear. There has been a suit, and expensive lawyers have been flown in from the North. The hospital lost. It plans to appeal and fly in more expensive lawyers from maybe even Further North. Administrative overhead soars, and it is no wonder that 26 percent of medical "care" costs are consumed by "administration."

"Why," I am often asked by my patients, "are hospital costs so high anyway?" In my generous spirited way, and feeling the allegiance I have always felt toward our institutions of health care, I have invariably risen to their defense.

"Well, we must remember they have just bought a new magnetic desuscitator, a cyclotron for the outpatient department, a particle accelerator and three complementary resonators for the surgical suite, laser dishwashers, and a new mahogany table for the board room. These things cost money, but," I say more brightly, "they will allow us to make a more rapid diagnosis in case you come down with a paniculoblastoma."[2] The patients, although invariably impressed, are quick to riposte their telling blow, "but it cost me $10 for a Kleenex." They then produce the bill as proof, wondering if there is anything I can do about it. It takes a lot to placate some people, after all, but I have given time and my best care to gentle assuagements.

In any case it is agreeable to believe and hope that consideration and compassion are cheap to dispense, and have positive meanings that can be weighed in the balance against high technology and the apotheosis of the budget. Not that I seriously advocate a return to horse and buggy medicine, though that may be in the offing too, come to think of auto exhaust and ozone pollution. And who knows, hard economics may force us all to do with less. Meanwhile, if we as a profession have been humbled by various social and bureaucratic forces, it is no reason for the hospitals to exalt themselves and go around economically credentialing everyone and getting sued and countersuing. It simply raises the cost of the Kleenex with which our patients perform their rhinophlegmectomies.

Surely there can be found better and more amiable ways to continue providing good medical care, lower the cost of Kleenex, and maintain the trust between hospital and physician. Perhaps some clever economist can in fact come up with a cheaper way to blow our noses, but suing the hard working and worthy physicians of one's staff is not the way to go about it.

Hospitals might recall, after all, that as their physicians we are their best asset and, indeed, don't even charge them for our services.

[2]To my knowledge no such tumor exists, but if it did it would be a vicious cancer of a primitive, that is to say very youthful, fat cell. Of course many of us, not so youthful at that, are constantly battling regular, old, fatty surfeit, particularly around the middle.

LETTER FROM THE MASKED MAN

lthough tending herein to limit myself to the personal and particular, I cannot help but feel impressed by a recent juxtaposition of events occurring Here and There.

By "Here," of course, I mean little old Tallahassee, right from the very heart of a hospital, which all of us for many years have held in great respect, granting to it our time and loyalty. Here, as that hospital struggles to cement its image of power upon our community and the medical profession, we have all been recently treated to a Media Spectacular. We have seen, in a series of five closely written articles in the local paper, revelations that the hospital is plagued by physicians who use its facilities (good grief!) to make a living! Let me quote from the hospital's legal brief so you clearly get the point, namely, that The Great Institution is "not a bus station" for physicians to use at their will for the treatment of patients!

As for the "There" I mean "Way Up There," but oh, so close, in Washington and Wall Street . . . The Journal in any case.

As I read an article in the *Wall Street Journal*, delivered to the door of my hotel room every morning while at a meeting of surgeons, it crossed my brainpan that, "Yessiree, if we physicians are going to survive Washington, we had better feel mighty comfortable in our relations with our local hospitals!"

What if, as this article foretold over the near horizon, the government indeed quits paying physicians for services rendered and, with grand largesse of manner, gratefully relinquishes that responsibility to the hands of your local hospital administrator?

Then, thought I, there will be a reckoning to conjure with, a haggling over nickels and dimes, and a hammering out of pennies between myself and the hospital. And how am I to have faith in negotiations with an institution capable of seeing its premium asset, an excellent staff of physicians, as a competitive threat?

Doubtless, I should then have to listen to heart-wrenching words as I am informed by the hospital of the economically desperate circumstances surrounding The Great Institution. Even worse, I will be forced to hear . . . and with what poor words of mine to counter? . . . the sincerity of The Great Institution's wish that they could do better for me; but times have now become so hard that for the surgery I have done on "their" patient they can, stretching it at that, allow me but two cents.

The door will close on that interview and what will be my recourse? Shall I seek redress by saving half my two cents and purchase a penny attorney to plead my case? Or shall I go hungry and get a full-fledged two-cent lawyer? And what difference will the two-cent one make against what seems the remarkable thousands of dollars that The Great Institution Here, and perhaps also in your particular There, appears to have available in spite of all to sue its own staff and support the legal profession?

Well, so what? We will still be physicians; the MD will, after all, still be back of our names.

It is at this point that the Letter from the Masked Man arrived, unsigned otherwise, and postmarked from a village up in Georgia. It was received by a large proportion of our physician population. The letter was a full, single-spaced page indicting physician naiveté in the face of the Machiavellian practices of Real Business, furthermore noting the writer's perception that physicians are "such a strange lot, incredibly naive about your strengths and weaknesses."

But let me quote at greater length this curious missive, so you get a feel for its interesting tone. It began: "Dear Medical Doctors: I read with a chuckle the recent *Tallahassee Democrat* articles on Tallahassee Memorial Regional Medical Center (TMRMC)'s policies on Doctors, Medical Staff membership, and business competition. I passed it off as silly until I met with my dear friend, my personal Doctor. I soon realized that he truly did not realize how we in the business world really operate. My dear friends, I hate to tell you this, but everything that the CEO [of the hospital] said is true. That attorney said it all, IT'S BUSINESS. Understand what that means for you. You are not a profession; you will be the worker bees. You will do what you are told or you will not play in their house. They will define how you work, where you work, when you work, and ultimately how you will get paid. Having been in the policy-making arm of the health industry, I am very familiar with their goals. Blame it on the doctors! They are the weakest politically and financially. Once they get control of the health-care dollar, you're theirs, PERIOD. And as weak as you all are politically (you really are a pitiful lot), you're really ripe for pluckin'. . . . How silly you are. I still can't believe my eyes when I read that paper. TMRMC is telling the patients that YOU are the cause of all the problems, YOU are the greedy ones, and the best line of all, the hospital exists to protect the patient from YOU."

With many specifics of local interest between, the letter ends "I don't hold out much hope for my dear old doc; he thinks different from me."

And so we do, I suppose, for we have not been trained for the world we find ourselves in.

But so what? Well, there are many "so whats" having to do with ideals and professionalism, autonomy and patient advocacy that you know as well as I to regret the loss of. Nor need I, even if I could, construct some essay wondering what indeed is a hospital these days? No longer is its definition merely a place where the sick are treated, but sadly sometimes more that of the "Big Place on the corner where Power and Control are out to reign supreme."

But again, "So what?" In our community, right now, such a concern seems neither here nor there except to us physicians and, at least in passing, the masked letter writer. It will be interesting to see if his forebodings for us prove true. And they very well may unless we perceive the urgency of our becoming as equal advocates for ourselves as we have traditionally been for our patients. We will, indeed, be best assisting them by the assertion of ourselves.

Up here in North Florida we need to do so this minute, because minutes in Tallahassee may be all we have before we find ourselves, sadly, neither Here nor There but in some Hereafter.

OVERVIEW: THE BREAST

One of the unsung pleasures of being a plastic surgeon, and more specifically a male plastic surgeon (subcategory: aesthetic surgeon of the female breast), is that one is spared by close professional association with this organ, so lovely in its shape and implications, many (if not all!) of those pangs and pains that otherwise must afflict the masculine male, and especially maybe the macho masculine male. Being something of an enthusiast of beautiful shapes, I feel a certain gratitude that I can regard a décolletage with a certain aesthetic detachment divorced from those maddening encumbrances that to some considerable measure fascinate and so tantalizingly rivet the attention of the susceptible gentleman.

This is not to say that I am "ho-hum" regarding the female breast. As a lovely aesthetic shape, in its ideal, fulfilling all those necessary architectural obbligatos of "form following function," and endowed with a rich history of cultural implication (by which I am bound to include down-home forthright eroticism) there is no bit of the human anatomy that compares with it.

The male phallus, by contrast I might note in passing, is a poor thing, without any pretense to elegance of contour, and should not be compared, though some have tried, to any sort of obelisk. D. H. Lawrence, of course, did his best to glamorize it and, as I recall from my youthful reading of that novel, made Lady Chatterly say all sorts of absurd things about it in the hope of rendering it more aesthetically acceptable. Her gardener-stud, quite full

of himself, gave it cute little nicknames, but which even to my teenage mentality patently failed to give this organ aesthetic credibility.

Be that as it may, I swear to you that the breast, beyond all of our organs,
is the most pop-idol-superstar of our anatomy. Even the heart, even the brain,
pales before it, neither almost ever appearing on the cover of *Cosmopolitan*
magazine, and how much less the ileum or jejunum. The naked male phallus,
or a heart or a brain, simply doesn't compare with the breast when it comes
to selling copy. In fact, there is something slightly "yucky" about most of our
organs that the breast, God bless it, has thoroughly escaped.

In any case, before getting more deeply into this flurry of essays, I want
to affirm that I am all for the breast. I am not, however, altogether
absolutely sure if it is my favorite organ, and curiously enough I have a lingering, sort of Edwardian penchant, perhaps inherited from my father, for
the ankle. Of course in his youth the breast was not much disclosed;
although it seems to me that those "Gibson Girls," though buttoned up to
the neck, suggested beneath their bouffant blouses a considerable thrilling
something. But in those times of yore, when "legs" had to be called "limbs"
in polite society, and no man had ever, perhaps, seen a female leg, the
glimpse of a shy ankle would be quite enough to cause something to happen
in one's "loin," as D. H. Lawrence persistently called it, wherever that is. My
father loved a good ankle, and I think even the foot connected; and so do I,
bless him. But I do not think an ankle, these days, would sell much copy on
the cover of *Cosmopolitan*, ours being such harder times.

I can remember the first breast I ever really saw, to lust after at least. I
was 14 and in prep school. The 15-year-old daughter of one of the masters,
who lived in a pretty white house just across a green from the dormitory
where we raunchy lads ate our Wheaties, would take breakfast with her
mom and dad in that same dining hall, where they, the parents, were sta-
tioned for breakfast themselves to keep us in some semblance of order. For
some reason the young lady was always a bit late. There were broad win-

dows through which, if you sat on the right side of the round table at which were seated perhaps eight of us, you would see her come bouncing across the green. She was pretty, and she was also precocious. Certainly she had an excellent mind. She was excellently endowed otherwise too. Those who got to look out the window paused as they brought their Wheaties-laden spoons to their mouths; she disappeared around a corner, and those who didn't get to look out the windows then got to watch her undulate, to us more of a ululation, across the dining room to join her parents. Our conversations would turn to saltpeter, although I was never sure quite what saltpeter did, or was in the first place; nor even how to spell it, and fruitlessly sought the right words to camouflage my ignorance. It seems to me, once, one of our stolid group, from New York City and therefore bristling with sophistication, noted learnedly that she was a "full C cup," and went on, seeing how excited the table became, to note that she "might even be a D." His very words, this "cup business," naturally caused our "loins" to ache.

Forgive me if I do not dwell here on the experience as it must have been perceived by the young lady herself. That is beyond my capability. I think, even at age 14, I sometimes wondered how she stood it. On the other hand I much more often thought she rather enjoyed it, and we were all of the philosophy that she arrived late specifically so she could wend her way among us lowly creatures, already seated before her arrival. Be that as it may, I extrapolate from this microcosmic experience to note that the poor male, smitten as he is in our culture by this bit of anatomy, must be looked upon . . . I beg of you . . . with some degree of kindness and generosity. Except for the occasional Don Giovanni amongst us, we are not permitted, after all, a very rich or extended examination of the female breast in its pristine glories. Oh, beaches being what they are, you may say, there are plenty of boobs out there to be ogled at; but this is not a particularly satisfactory solution, and is certainly unfulfilling.

The sad fact is that the male, in our culture, is trained from an early point to regard the female breast as a starving man might regard steak and potatoes. It is dangled before us everywhere. It is on the screen, it is smeared all over the TV set, it is on every magazine in the check-out line at the grocery store, and calendars announce a new pair with every month. And the shapes of those thus displayed, for delectation or sales purposes, are invariably the most exquisite examples. And yet, alas!, it is only to be seen, and never, ever, to the last degree, touched!

And yet, think I, how many men, good men and true, restraining themselves, go through life thus everywhere so keenly tempted, but remain . . . allow me here a trumpet fanfare . . . gentlemen!

Now, please, allow me to observe that I did not choose to go into plastic surgery in even any least little degree contemplating the fact that I would have the opportunity to view, and to touch, if you may call it that, legions of female breasts. Had I based any such decision on such crass and craven needs, I might, recognizing my slight penchant for the ankle, have gone into podiatry. Even so, I have now dealt with a very large number of breasts, and I feel thankful for it. To have done so has spared me that salient lusting after this organ that I think many men must endure. I have seen all forms of breasts, all shapes and sizes. I have helped people, and indeed they are grateful whichever way you go, by making them bigger, or by making them smaller. I have balanced things up. I have shored up the sags of motherhood. I have reconstructed the breast missing following ablation for cancer. Like the airplane pilot, who yet we hope may know and love the thrills of flight, I have done it enough so that I do not have to be intimidated by the circumstance.

There is something rather pleasant about knowing that beneath that elegant blouse, heaving or not, I can pretty closely predict the contour, and need not as a result agitate my imagination. I never ever gape at a lady's breast, because my practiced eye, in the least millisecond, comes to a complete understanding of the finest details, and I can quite engage myself with the lady's eyes, or her wit, or her pleasant intelligence. No more than when you meet a psychiatrist, and think he is analyzing you when he is absolutely not, do I need to be introduced to a breast, and make a fool of myself falling into it.

This, I say to you, is one of the pleasant, if relatively minor, prerogatives of the practicing male plastic surgeon. I share it with you because I am not certain that these points have ever been noted before . . . .

Beyond which the following spate (not untouched with spite) of essays will note my offense that this opulent titbit . . . choosing herewith the unbowdlerized term over the more prudish Victorian "tidbit" . . . which replaced it . . . of anatomy was so shamelessly preyed upon in the Great Silicone Breast Debacle of 1991. No study has ever demonstrated any relationship between silicone and any disease, either before or since. Even the FDA now agrees, even that most scientific of journals, *Science*, says as much.[1] But, capitalizing on the understandable fear of ladies regarding the health of their breasts, an unfeeling and unthinking media, combining that fear with the fascination intrinsic to this organ, marched into the living rooms of 2 million ladies to terrify them. I have, myself, never yet seen a lady made ill from her silicone or any other implant; but certainly I saw innumerable ladies, perfectly happy and with excellent results, tortured and made hysterical by the allegations the media, and I might add the legal community, presumed to terrify them with.

Well, the media and the lawyers might say, "Why blame us?" We live in a world where all is fair game, and to overlook the potential of such a lovely and lurid mix of Death and Beauty, of which high drama after all is made, would be merely to lose a great opportunity.

So be it. And yet, just perhaps, it is worth noting in perspective that this issue, so beautifully and thrillingly orchestrated, entailed a set of circumstances respecting which—unlike what one might say of aspirin, penicillin, bees, and the automobile—no one to my knowledge, even allegedly, has

[1] *Science*, 11 Dec. 1998, volume 282, number 5396, p.1963.

ever died of. In fact, for what it is worth, I read a newspaper article once describing the most fortuitous titbit of good luck when, in a club of some sort, one of the female dancers was accidentally shot by a random bullet. She was, very happily, struck in the breast, which being partly made of silicone absorbed the impact and, in fact thereby, saved her life.

It makes me thoughtful regarding the possibilities for those ladies who serve with our front-line troops, or as members of "the thin blue line," standing so gallantly between ourselves and mayhem.

BRANDY, PLEASE, A DOUBLE

I sometimes think it would be comforting, within reason of course, to be a harder drinking man. I have always vaguely marveled at those people in movies, often enough cowboys, not unusually detectives, but even rarely physicians, who, when the going gets tough, seem so comforted by a "stiff drink" tossed down. As for myself I will occasionally have a martini on the rocks, but mostly as a vehicle for filling a sparkling martini glass with olives and ice, and settling down after a hard day and a shower to impress my wife with my debonair manners and means.

On the occasion, however, of some interesting news from Dow Corning, erstwhile silicone-supplier to the world, stronger stuff was called for, like whiskey neat mixed with a bottle of Wry.

At present, forgive me that I have not much in the way of specifics, but (as the story itself quite demonstrates) in our world what difference are "facts" when barely informed speculation is so much more thrilling? As Oscar Wilde quite neatly put it, he felt no need to prejudice his opinion in the review of a literary work by actually reading it.

In any case, it is a quite sufficient fact, if not one that is going to drive me to wretched drink, that Dow Corning has in the blandest possible manner, so bland as to barely reach the back pages of the news, attempted to buy off the silicone-breast-implant-containing public with a proposal to divvy up almost 5 Billion (that's a capital "b") to those silicone-implanted ladies possessing any one of a rather grand list of symptoms. I have not seen the list of diagnoses, but some fatuous source says that hemorrhoids may be on it and why not, let us hope, bad hair days and "the Blahs." All it will take to get a chunk of this loot will be for one, single, solitary, not even sober physician to vouch for the fact that one of the designated symptoms exists in the implanted (breast only) patient.

First of all, of course, it is marvelous to think of all the people who may thus readily get this lot of money for having had an operation with which they may have been quite pleased, even if now it putatively causes hemorrhoids. Perhaps better, especially to the red-blooded American physician, is the wry possibility, if not indeed intent, of Dow Corning to cut out the lawyers altogether. To get your piece of these billions, it is specifically mentioned that the negotiation can be performed without the least presence of legal counsel. Well, we shall see about that, but for the present, anyway, it is a delectable dish to think of the attorneys salivating over such monies floating around from which they, for heavens' sake, might be excluded! Have you ever heard the like?

But let me not wallow in pleasant images. If by this method of payoff Dow Corning can excuse itself from any complaint, nuisance, or suit whatsoever in perpetuum forever and after, more power to them; after all, the legal community has in reserve another pot of gold, as yet essentially unmined, of the plastic surgeons themselves. Yes, there have been some incredible awards to individuals who have undergone breast augmentation, but as yet none of these have named the surgeons in any particular fashion, most being content with what has been extractable from the business community and manufacturers. I am, myself, ready for anything, recognizing grimly that a time may come when I may have to start putting more gin than olives in my martini.[1]

But never mind my simple expostulations and amazements. I am too prone to these, and we need to look at this offer in sterner fashion.

---

[1]Miraculously, such has not occurred, which leads me to have a more sanguine attitude towards the legal profession, even though I am putting a little more gin in my martini anyway, just to be on the safe side.

First of all, for those of you who not so avidly followed the affairs of silicone as a debacle, I would like to note that there is as yet no valid scientific evidence that silicone causes any sort of disease whatsoever, certainly nothing that caught anyone's attention for 35 years of fairly close study and use, nor in the last few years of intensive, almost frantic on occasion, effort. The subtleties of the disease process and what may trigger it remain ultimately a bit obscure for any disease whatsoever. One can accordingly scarcely say with absolute certainty that silicone is "safe," or at least safer than getting out of bed every morning, or for that matter safer than staying in bed continuously. It may be that indeed someone out there somewhere has some sort of predisposing genetic or immunological circumstance that silicone acting mysteriously as some form of adjuvant may trigger. No one argues that patients deserve the best elaboration they can be given of these statistics and mechanisms, if such can be discovered.

So much for sense and science. On the other hand, how wondrous it is that we get to live in an age where the mere threat of suit can result in the extortion offered up in hopeful sacrifice of $5 billion. Yet calculating boardroom brains clearly decided this offer would be, after all, the better business decision compared to the expense, worry, tedium, and final costs of being picked at for 10 or 20 years by plaintiffs' attorneys. We all know how insurance companies may settle despite a defendant's innocence for a few tens of thousands of dollars, or even hundreds, to save themselves from being picked to the bone by the hyenas of the judicial process; but $5 billion surely is a record.

Surely, also, the record breaks marvelous new ground in the vindication of "junk science." The clever orchestration of quarter truths, and outright lies, dating from the 1988 pronouncement of Sidney Wolfe, speaking from his pulpit as the Director of the Medical Branch of "Public Citizen," that silicone causes breast cancer, has led us step by hysterical step to this interesting juncture. If plastic surgery has been belittled, the means by which this has occurred deserves the scrutiny of every physician, and better controls over how scientific evidence, or lack of it, may be presented in the courtroom. If the syringes used by diabetics contain silicone as a lubricant, why is this fact not much dwelt upon? As has been well said, this was really not so much a "silicone" but rather a "breast" issue.

But $5 billion! I stand in awe of the figure. It is as many dollars as the amount of time in years since our planet began to coalesce from its amorphous, molten origins. It is half the amount of time since the Big Bang and the beginning of the universe. From a more pragmatic perspective, I recall reading of Congress struggling as it debated the issue of whether to assist Russia with a $1.5 billion aid package. It is clear that Russia would have been much better off negotiating with Dow Corning. I am forced to conclude that we live in a marvelous, wonderful country where magic and wizardry still can work their spells.

But wait! Will $5 billion be enough? After all, 1.5 million pairs of implants, not even counting lawyers, divided into $5 billion is only $33,333.33. Compared to the $17 million recently awarded by a trial jury, it is paltry pittance!

Maybe I will have a dry martini, and easy on the olives too!

TO WASHINGTON!
LIKE MR. SMITH I WISH

I have in mind that the FDA must logically ban the automobile. You may think I'm not being serious, so let me emphasize that I always am and quite earnestly so in this instance. We need to get rid of this automobile "thing," which I hereby propose to prove is a more deadly apparatus than, yes, the silicone implant. First, despite odds and ends of piecemeal testing, the automobile was never properly studied by appropriate government agencies. It was—terrible mistake—simply "grandfathered" in and has since killed, maimed, and left destitute more than, as we are wont to say, all our wars put together plus saccharine.

It seems clear to me that the FDA should at least demand of General Motors, Ford, and the others that there be produced not merely retrospective but prospective studies, perfectly conforming to the Bureau of Protocol Standards, plus thousands of pages of data to demonstrate the safety of this noxious vehicle over the horse.

On the other hand, why not ban it outright, saying to hell with statistics, because it does seem reasonably clear, if one must allow reason, that for numerous years almost 50 thousand people have been killed annually by this machine? Nor let us forget the 2 or 3 million variously incapacitated and put out of work at great cost to their family's and our country's economic well-being. Furthermore, need I remind you, the automobile is an ecological disaster, contributing even more to depletion of the ozone layer than hair spray and bovine flatus.

Let me mobilize more than merely rational facts. I offer the modest suggestion that reason be laced liberally with hysteria, this deed accomplished by the simple expedient of introducing the topic to the media. By so doing the issue will instantly become "political," generating more hysterics, and with unpredictable consequences to our ozone layer because politics is even more gaseous than cows.

What about the more subtle diseases caused by automobiles? Who, for example, has not had the experience of "nodding off" on a long tedious journey, driving late at night? If so, can it be denied that the automobile is a pretty clear cause of what most properly could be called "chronic fatigue syndrome"? I once almost went over a vast precipice when afflicted by this condition, and was rendered not only hysterical but for many months my autoimmune system felt tangibly depleted.

I ask you, what kind of government do we live under that allows such a device to run amuck among its citizenry, killing, injuring, and rendering hysterical so many, while at the same time poisoning the very air we breathe?

I don't mean to sound shrill; rather I want to be thoughtful, reasonable, and balanced. On the other hand, it is difficult for me not to twitch and froth; nay, rend the air, when I think of how the tragic, innocent little silicone implant, made of the veritable stuff that is the baseline standard for all other implant materials, is being hounded by our huge government, which seems much more apt to take its evidence from Connie Chung and the media than from the balanced experience and interpretation of 30 years of data. Besides, implanting silicone is an ecologically sound operation that has proven itself over the 20 years that I have been doing it as quite easily the safest, happiest, and most positive of any I do in terms of the patient's relationship to our world. Must it be wantonly maligned by committees who still allow themselves the choice to smoke cigars?

If they ban the implant, perhaps they should also legislate separate restaurant seating areas for "ladies with silicone."

Well, I am answering the call. My society has put out a plea that we unite and march on Washington in defense of this little artifact which, more than any medical device I know, has a still sweetness and positive beauty that inspires a muttered exclamation, something like Keats: "Thou still unravished bride of quietness . . ."

Yes, even I, most modest in habit and practice, shall gird on some sort of aging armor and sally forth to attempt a meeting with sensible senators and humbly joust. I will try to sound like James Stewart when he went to Washington Hollywood style. Everything came out all right then. I will entreat them, if they permit the automobile, to cease this senseless regulation of kinder and gentler options, limiting drastically, in this instance, "women's choice."

Even now insurance companies, ever alert, are on the verge of denying 2 million ladies coverage for breast disease of any sort if there is the sniff of silicone about them. Two million ladies, indeed, are on the threshold of becoming second class citizens. All this despite the fact that no study yet known shows any scientific or rational evidence of harm done, but in the vast majority only happiness. It is, begging your forbearance, a quality-of-life issue, and are we not advocates of this for our patients?

What, by the way, shall we cover pacemakers with, or make catheters and drains of, or joint replacement prostheses? It will be the end of that business for Dow Corning, the only manufacturer of medical-grade silicone and silastic in our country. Who will inherit the world market? The Japanese, of course, the only other world manufacturer, who will be glad for us to export yet another chunk of our economy to theirs.

Furthermore, I shudder but delight to ask, why is there no fine hoopla over silicone testicular implants for the well-dressed gentleman? Someone in Washington needs to be kicked in them, I humbly submit.

Let me reassure you, however, I do promise to be discreet in our Capital and bear myself thus wisely so that you, the reader, will be proud.

{ *NOLO NOCERE* }

Since the advent of the media extravaganza surrounding the silicone implant, I have been pondering life and, in it, how "safe" must be "safe"?

Forgive me, yet again, for mentioning *implantum siliconium;* every time I write this word I swear never to again, but face it, this is the most intense media issue I have ever dealt with medically. Even though the issue may be distant from your own interest, as a fiendish perpetration, it demonstrates how vulnerable we presently are in the practice of medicine.

But never mind this erstwhile pleasant little device for the moment.

Ponder marbles instead: While reading the paper the other day I saw that after hot contention, a considerable bureaucratic commission finally arrived at the conclusion that marbles measuring over 1.6 cm in diameter will not have to conform to a proposed requirement that each be stamped with words to the effect "This marble could be dangerous to your health." I was thrilled to hope that a breath of fresh air and common sense might have been interjected into the due and serious deliberations of those authorities in Washington who are eager to oversee our safety.

I realize, of course, that marbles can be risky business. I remember when I was 12 years old shooting a few of them at other fellows with sling shots, and I once knew a child who swallowed one, but without incident after they caught it at the other end a few days later, and he was all right. On the other hand, every now and then a kid chokes on one. Perhaps kids should be warned against this potential, but a marble, after all, simply does not have enough surface area to describe on it all the dangers potential to its hard, shiny, compelling, and colorful roundness.

Perhaps each could come packaged with a "manufacturer's insert," describing the dire effects properly, and in large print, too, that a seven-year-old could eagerly read. But I grow ridiculous, and prefer at this moment simply to praise the government's common sense on this issue, at least.

But very seriously, how "safe" must be "safe"?

Dr. David Kessler, chief factotum of the FDA, allowed a couple of months ago to the news media that a role of the physician is to "do no harm." This is a noble sentiment, particularly when said in Latin, and is a precept we bow before. Even so, when he said it, in somewhat fine and sanctimonious fettle before a field of cameras, I could not repress an involuntary frisson and luffing of my sails. If safety is to be an absolute virtue, very little could be permitted; and if some things are permissible, by what criteria can committees come to conclusions that the pleasure of playing marbles, for example, outweighs the risk? In the absence of "criteria" we are left with Bias, Media Coverage, Politics, Money, Power, Ego, Law, and what is Politically Correct.

Carrying these ruminations to the happy absurd, I had a pleasant fantasy the other day while holding pressure onto something bleeding . . . five minutes by the clock. I cast myself in the role of a news reporter. I saw myself at a press conference being given by, why not say a Dr. K (the "K" made famous by Kafka) in his role as Commissioner for Public Safety? I imagined the Commissioner as having just placed a "moratorium" on the selling, serving, or in any way eating of red meats. I conceived that fish and chicken would be for the present excluded from this ban, but that these were to undergo separate investigations at further expensive hearings later in the year. My daydream continued . . . .

"But chicken and fish," said Dr. K, "also may represent a clear and present danger to the American public, because both contain bones conducive to choking or enlodgement within a Zenker's diverticulum."[1] He paused for serious effect, because part of his job description is to be mostly particularly "serious." "Right now we are focusing our attention on Steak-House Syndrome, which results in the death of a significant number of Americans every year, with serious injuries related to broken ribs and ruptured bowels resulting from the injudicious application of the Heimlich maneuver. As a matter of fact, once we have finished with chicken and fish, we will be convening a panel of psychologists, vegetarians, and homeopaths to give us their advice regarding banning, as well, the Heimlich maneuver itself for the reasons aforementioned."

Once the hub-hub settled down following the Commissioner's remarks, my colleagues in the press arose to ask him the usual pointed questions:

Q: "In your estimation, Dr. K, is there a place here, in a free society, to allow 'choice'? I mean, Sir, if every restaurant and food server were to explain the complications of beef eating, would this be sufficient reason to allow beef to remain on the market?"

Dr. K: "The answer is 'No' to the first part of your question and 'No' to the second. Next question please."

Q: "Sir, what advice would you give the beef-eating portion of the American public regarding the high levels of cholesterol, preservatives, fatty acids, blood, splinters of bone, and trace elements of cyanide, silicone, and slow viruses that are found in beef?"

Dr. K: "It is my suggestion they rush to their lawyer for advice. Next question please."

Q: "Given the known incidence of Death-By-Peanut Syndrome, when a nut is tossed in the air and caught in the mouth by the victim, aspirated by him/her with almost immediate death, what is your position on the peanut?"

---

[1] A troublesome outpouching in the esophagus, where all manner of debris can collect and foment, causing mischief.

Dr. K: "We will shortly be doing in-depth studies of the peanut. As you know, we have roomfuls of data regarding its lethal potential, and I might add that I have just come into possession of what we shall call the so-called 'Secret Memos' from Planter's, which suggested that they have known all along that peanuts cause cancer." An aide leaned over towards Dr. K, whispering into his ear. "Oh, sorry," he went on, "I was a little confused there, and am informed that I am mixing up the peanut with silicone. But probably Planter's does have that evidence somewhere . . . it's just that the peanut is not as sexy as silicone . . . and . . ." his voice trailed off.

The press conference over, I rushed out with my buddies, and we all had a steak and some peanuts for lunch, and a touch of simethicone trisilicate[2] for dessert.

The bleeding in my patient had long stopped. "Eureka," I thought to myself, "another perfect result safely performed," etc.

That evening I had an actual martini with four olives, mulling over how the juniper berry had curiously yet escaped the oversight of our bureaucracy, and glad the olives did not contain those dangerous, marble-like seeds, but only soft pimento.

Afterward, I felt balmy and forgiving, a kind of "there-there" feeling that permitted me to allow that Dr. K was doing the best he could, in a difficult job, plagued by his own fears and prejudices. What more, surrounded by the fast machines that drive our moment, can one do?

Maybe not much.

But maybe I, at least, shall start to play more marbles. A grand game, you know, and pretty safe too. The government has almost said so!

---

[2] A popular antacid containing something of silicone.

THE DEFENSE RESTS,
WITH FOOTNOTES[1]

I tend these days to be suddenly somber, by fits and starts; sometimes even serious, hmmmmm-ing a good deal.[2]

Outwardly I am altogether calm, decently humored, and interested in the weather. We have had much rain and pleasantly at night, with our bedroom windows open, its sound is heard "dripping from the eaves and bells of flowers"[3] amongst the ivy and the "twisted eglantine."[4] I take our nine-year-old daughter on Monday nights to her harp lessons, for which good purpose I miss our local medical society meetings, preferring her music to "gin and beer,"[5] although I miss the oysters.[6] I drink no more than my usual four martinis a week, but note that I am lately putting three olives on the toothpick, one eaten immediately, one in *media res*, and a final for "dessert" after which we dine elegantly by candlelight, *en famille*, on pasta or potatoes. To Miss Meredith, of the aforementioned harp, I have just completed reading aloud *Treasure Island*[7] and now for bedtime recreation we are commencing *Swallows and Amazons*.[8] This litany of "devices" I only note for the sake of

---

[1]As defined by the fact of a lengthy mess of footnotes, and in case on the witness stand they ask me "if I have written any scientific articles lately?"

[2]See "Hmm" under "Homely."

[3]Stevens, Wallace, an American insurance executive with a poetical flare, 1879–1955.

[4]Milton, John: "L'Allegro," 1608–1674.

[5]Kipling, Rudyard, as in "You may talk of . . ."; sued twice in America, 1865–1936.

[6]Carroll, Lewis: "The Walrus and the Carpenter," 1832–1898.

[7]Stevenson, R.L., 1850–1894, author and would-be pirate.

[8]Ransome, Arthur, ca. 1930, another pirate want-to-be.

their "homeliness" and what I might also call "good"; that, as you may note above, is after all two-thirds of what this book is about.

Then there is the "Bad."

Permit me accordingly to subtitle this particular "essay" (in quotes because I do not want to do that lovely literary form any rude injustice) "Silicone Implants Part IV." Actually it might be Part "V," but that's not the kind of information I am much troubling myself about these days.

What does trouble me is how I shall respond to "The Summons" if and when it occurs from, of course, that source of all "Summonses," namely the Great and Veritable Dignity of the Law.[9]

For the present I note that I am seeing my patients with an almost fiercely acute awareness of the privilege they have done me in trusting me with their bodies, usually to have put upon themselves some sort of scar delivered *de novo* by myself or repaired as best I can post-traumatic injury. My patients seem a dash transfigured in my eye as an almost spiritual resource. As Dr. Johnson[10] said, the imminence of hanging wonderfully concentrates a man's thoughts and in this silicone implant business, never minding that it has been the safest and happiest operation of my professional life, one discovers now the long shadow of the gibbet.

It goes something like this. Awakening at 1:00 A.M., I hear the rain falling, a blessing to the ear and upon the heads of small frogs. My level of consciousness rising, I begin to make a mental effort not to think but to simply revel in the sound of the rain and on Thursday nights "the cool kindliness of (clean) sheets,"[11] my wife's warm toes, and the sweet scent of whatever sachet is in her chest of drawers lingering yet about her nightgown. In spite of all I become more widely awake. I try the exercise my wife has taught me.

---

[9]Coke, Sir Edward, 1552–1634; Bean, Judge "Hanging" Roy, late 19th century.
[10]Johnson, Dr. Samuel, not "Billy," 1709–1784.
[11]Brooke, Rupert, 1887–1915. "The Great Lover"; Thursday being the day we change our bed linens.

Pick a word and run through its letters in sequence, trying to think of the names of every artist?, baseball player?, fish?, or whatever category, that I can recall beginning with each letter. The other night she even gave me my word, "turnip." The exercise worked. I did Turner[12] and Tiepolo,[13] skipped "u" and went directly to "r," peeling off "Rembrandt"[14] and curiously "Romney,"[15] and was back asleep. On some occasions I am simply too petulant, won't play the game at all, and so get into moiling, broiling, bubbling, and boiling.[16]

With the implants "off the market" it is simply a kind of bitter pill to see my patients in follow up; all suddenly seem perfect, soft, thrilled, their lives enhanced, and scarcely any now making little whimpering noises about wishing they were "bigger." The silicone implant loss reminds me of Napoleon haranguing his troops before the Sphinx, "men, history is looking down upon you"[17]; of happy options now "Gone With the Wind"[18]; of "where are the snows of yesteryear"[19]; and of all things that have been a touch of magic, now flown forever away.

Never mind these sentiments; there are harder matters with which we must deal, and which may well intend to deal with us.

If you happen to be someone who in your career has put a touch of silicone into anyone, there is, I fear, the potential of being brought rudely to account. True, just now the sharks are circling the manufacturer of silicone, Dow Corning, setting the stage for a fine feeding frenzy. When that carcass is left bare-boned, will not their insatiable eyes look elsewhere for flesh to

---

[12]Turner, not "Ted," but J.M.W., 1775–1851.
[13]As in Tiepolo, G.B., 1696–1770, not the rock star.
[14]As in Rembrandt van Rijn, 1606–1669, not Jones.
[15]Romney, G. (not his brother if he had one), 1734–1802.
[16]What finally happened to MacBeth.
[17]Napoleon I, bashing about in Egypt, "Soldiers, 17 centuries look down upon you!"
[18]Like in the movie.
[19]Villon, François: 1431, early French insurance salesman, as in "Where are the snows of yesteryear?"

render? I tend to think it likely (or is this mere cynicism?) that we may plead our innocence and the quality of our care; that we may produce records that demonstrate the gratitude and joy our patients have expressed; that we may say there is no "scientific evidence" of ill effect, or if some is suddenly discovered that we never knew of it at the time of surgery. I fear, however, the law has its own means of legally devouring those it finds fit to consume.

On a personal note, and here is where I wish to get grandly dramatic and hope you will applaud me for it, I wonder if I should simply tear up the first letter from a lawyer wishing to sue me or only the fourth letter, because my liability coverage will provide some pale defense on the first three letters within any given year. I am tempted to tear up the first. Perhaps I might write a letter to the lawyer telling him I tore it up, that he could immediately go to Hell, and that I intend to see myself in chains[20] before I will play his blithe game (their letters are always so disinterested, so blandly detached) and thrown into prison for contempt of court rather than engaging myself in any way. I wonder what would happen? In my melodramatic way, I see the sheriff arriving at our house on a Monday night before I take my daughter to harp and dragging me off after reading me my "rights."

As you stand before a judge, what would happen if you said, "I do not wish to be a part of this whatsoever. Your due process is a travesty and an insult to my 25 years of caring for patients."[21]

Would they simply throw you in jail[22] and by neat (legal) means subsume all your assets to the plaintiff and the lawyer? I don't think they can take

[20]Lovelace, not Linda, but Richard, 1618–1657, as in "Stone walls do not a prison make . . . ."
[21]Obsolete, early English and American, now replaced by "clients," "subscribers," and "consumers."
[22]If so, and jails are suddenly overcrowded with physicians, what then, other than letting out the drug dealers and murderers to make room for us?

your home,[23] but maybe they can. Maybe they would make you do a million hours of "community service" which seems a popular sentence for miscreants. What if you said, "I've already done a million hours of 'community service,' in the emergency room on poor, battered folks who don't know what hit them," while the judge and lawyers sleep in their beds, awakening to give themselves yearly *pro bono* awards duly praised by the media.

It is clear to me that I will not be very able to deal with the sudden appearance of 10 or 20 or 50 suits. I am, accordingly in the wee hours of the night, pondering drastic and dramatic methods and turns of phrase. Forgive me if, herein, I practice on you, complete with their footnotes.

And, damn, I may even go see a friend, a trial lawyer for heaven's sake!, and hear what he thinks of my fantasies. I just hope he doesn't turn upon me a bland eye and a soothing tone . . . .

[23]Tim Warfel, my very own estate attorney, who implied to me that they can take everything IF you live in the city on something more than the one quarter acre that defines a "homestead." The lawyer may accordingly possess most of your house, living in the better rooms, while the plaintiff and her loud children have your old bedroom. You and your family are either under a tree or in a closet if it is raining.

AFTERVIEW: THE BREAST

Since these essays were written in the early nineties, numerous studies have been performed to the purpose of delineating what, if any, dangers may reside in the implantation of silicone in the human body. None have discovered any evidence that a lady with silicone implants is more at risk of developing disease, particularly those diseases of connective tissue with which they were allegedly associated, than any other person *sans* silicone. The most recent of these studies, reported in a December 1998 issue of the prestigious journal, *Science*, corroborates those findings. So too does the FDA.

I wonder: Do the law courts that awarded such remarkable sums to this issue ever wonder at themselves? Do they ever query the mechanisms implicit in our judicial system that so permit drama and the manipulation of anecdotal evidence to preside over common sense and reason? Can they resurrect the six or seven companies that, because of this great debacle, were forced into bankruptcy? Should money be ladled out before truth is ascertained?

Well, to be fair, out of this have come certain judicial requirements related to the quality of "expert testimony," which one hopes may in the future prevail. As for pain caused, and economic loss, the deed is, however, done. We do, after all, move forward, and none can be too critical if we do so confusedly as, wishing for the best, we live amongst anomaly, recalcitrant facts, greed, politics, prejudice, and fear.

Perhaps, as I tell my patients contemplating breast augmentation, the spasm is over, the issue pretty much settled. In the same breath I also tell

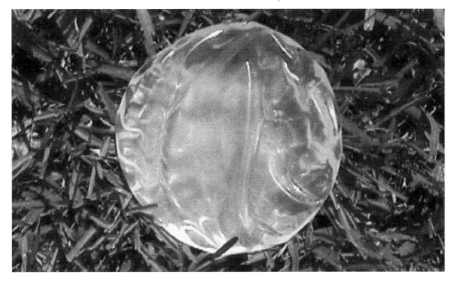

Silicone implant making mischief in our backyard.

them to be wary, arming them with such supportive facts as I can give them against what I guess may also be some new round that will contrive to make of the female breast an issue. It is simply too delectable an organ to be left quietly to itself and plastic surgeons. It contains within it too much of Beauty and Power almost equally mixed with Death and Disease. It has "grown up," and has become Big Business, almost to a point where it might as well be listed on the New York Stock Exchange. And business being business (*see* Letter from the Masked Man) there are naturally entrepreneurs who will be happy in its manipulation to make their own fortunes, and never mind pale guidelines as to expert testimony and rational evidence.

As Keats said, "Beauty is truth, truth beauty," and let me hope here that his opinion will prevail. It seems to me on the whole it contrives to do so; and meanwhile, if in the previous essays I have said things that sound cynical, or offended those who may be yet suffering, I sincerely apologize. I do not know much. But I do know that when people believe they are ill, afflicted by pain and fear, they deserve . . . no matter what I think or maybe know or probably know not . . . my greatest respect and compassion.

VEGETABLES AND OTHER MEDIA ALTERNATIVES

U p here, or down if you live in Georgia or the far north like
Tennessee, we are in the throes of "media coverage." Our
local newspaper has been enjoying an eruption of revelations
regarding the ill will existing, like electrical sparks, between
physicians and one of our major hospitals.

This "ill will" . . . its causes, ramifications, permutations, claims and con-
frontations . . . has given our local "investigative reporters" an opportunity
to sharpen their skills. Does it surprise you that we physicians have come
out just barely better than silicone?

As the volcanic spewings from this media extravaganza settle upon us, perhaps we can feel lucky, if not content, with no more than a final extra shovel-
ful of ash tossed upon our heads.

And so tossed a senior editor of our local newspaper, who seized upon the
latter-day physician to write a reminiscence of his own excellent grandfather,
a good, old-fashioned, "horse-riding country doctor," who lived with a full
beard "in the tiny town of Stanton, Kentucky." The editorial came complete
with a charming picture of this gentleman who looked remarkably like Abraham Lincoln.

The editorialist elaborated on his granddad's circumstances, allowing that he
had some money worries, which ultimately drove him to founding a bank. On
the other hand, and in the next breath of his essay, our editor noted that regarding the economic circumstance of the modern physician "there are so many other
rewards (in medicine) that money shouldn't even be close to the major one."

Quite true. He is right there. Good for him. I don't myself think it is "close to the major one," but just like grandpa we have to survive, but few of us in these vastly more complex social and bureaucratic times can found a bank. If the old grandpa was allowed difficulty making ends meet, is it fair to deny us, or anyone else, that possibility? Besides, let me note, our utility bills are infinitely higher than his granddad's, who may have had none, and particularly nowadays when you have a house full of 9-year-olds and teenagers who keep the air conditioning set constantly on "Antarctic." The old docs didn't have to put up with this sort of thing. They just opened the windows. Furthermore, they didn't have to pay taxes, social security, or beyond their wildest imaginings "malpractice premiums." For them, I think, "overhead" was not much more than the hay it took to feed the horse. Even so, our editor continues, "it is clear that doctors today don't have to accept a mess of greens as bill payment." The implication is pretty obvious that physicians today are fairly mean-spirited when it comes to reimbursement for services rendered.

We have heard all this before, and yet I wonder what it is in the public awareness that insists on equating "accepting a mess of greens," and presumably other vegetables as payment signifies that you are a good doctor: kind, compassionate, humanitarian, six feet two like the granddad, and with the flowing beard of a gentle patriarch. We are doubtless a profession unique in the public's determination that we should, after all is said and done, be perfectly content with a sack of vegetables in return for lithotripting a renegade ureteral calculus.

Yet I have (and doubtless most physicians otherwise) been content with just that for my services. Up here not only do I accept vegetables and eggs, but being near the great oyster beds of Apalachicola I have received quite a few quarts of oysters in compensation, an emolument I consider qualitatively superior, so long as they don't have some dreadful hepatitis lurking in their valves. Oysters are better than vegetables because you can have them with a beer, if you like, or even with a nip of chilled vodka, on a saltine cracker, with hot vinegar-sauce also given you by a patient, or a more prosaic dash of lemon juice. Anyone would work for that. Lacking oysters in Kentucky, where the old grandfather-doctor practiced, I can see why he would ultimately get disgusted with carrots, greens, and beans and take to founding banks. Implicit, nonetheless, is the clear fact that even for his venerableness vegetables did not quite cut it for him either.

Yet clearly, and in the best tradition, vegetable compensation to the MD is alive and well. I have marked as "paid" accounts of patients who have brought in greens, washed seven times (one has to be grateful for that!). I have been the happy recipient of corn on the cob, a case of peanut butter, two cases of pickles, a case of pickled okra once, untold bushels of tomatoes, and rather recently my first bag of potatoes. I have also received numerous bottles of pepper-vinegar, which goes well with the oysters if not the peanut butter, bushels of figs, dozens of eggs, and piles of peanuts, which, in case you have a wart you want removed, I prefer boiled.

But never mind such facts, which are merely seen from my own very homely and particular perspective, and may do your own attitudes an injustice.

It seems to me that the larger issue threatening us is that we physicians may stand on the brink of finding ourselves within that unprivileged circle of media peeves, rather like England's Royal Family, which I sometimes think the press will not leave alone until it is hounded to destruction. It may simply suit the media's present mood to trumpet against physicians making as good a living as we have been allowed in the past, and insisting that we conform to a more "politically correct" image, which reduces our professional definition to that of the merest trade, at the beck and call of administrators, bureaucrats, politicians, the legal profession, and other lesser vegetables.

Meanwhile, I continue to be happy to accept in payment most edibles, understanding full well the privilege and "other rewards" inherent in my profession. I can do so, on the other hand, only so long as I can keep a degree of independence, autonomy, dignity, and sufficient currency of the realm to pay my overhead, liability premium, mortgage, nurses and administrative staff, and the air conditioning bill. The problem, of course, is that none of the banks I deal with, nor my liability insurance carrier, nor for that matter anyone else I know, very happily accepts vegetables for their compensation. Do, I wonder, news editors?

Yet I still can. Just a couple of weeks ago I received a large plastic bag full of vegetables, which stayed in our office refrigerator for a few days, forgotten . . . or maybe I knew I could not take them home because the children, preferring Cheetos and potato chips, would have thrown rocks at me. But today, indeed only an hour before writing this, came along an old patient of mine, be-bopping down the sidewalk, and popping in unannounced to show me how beautifully his burn scar had matured over these past 12 years. He was a cheery note in my day. We had a pleasant reunion, filled with mutual compliments. He asked if I had a Coke I could give him to drink as he walked along. Yes indeed. I gave him not only a cold Coke, but a package of "Ry-Chee."

And also the bag of vegetables, a little limp but still good. I hope he enjoys them. He seemed thrilled. Thus happily doth the world turn. Thus gladly am I yet allowed to be a physician, in spite of editorial disparagements . . . and, dare I hint it, misconceptions.

ABOVE THE LAW

One thing I have recently noticed about Death is that, once you are there, even a lawyer cannot ring you up.

Because I was quite alive before Christmas, never mind my wildness of eye and a mild seasonal headache, I was accordingly available to all telephone appeals. It was not a lawyer, however, but a Doctor X somewhere up in Georgia who called.

"Oh dear," I thought to myself, "someone has ruptured her silicone implant that I put in years ago, silicone has flooded her system, gotten into her brain and knee joints, and caused failure to thrive in her nursing infant, who has suddenly lost all traces of extraocular motion and is staring fixedly at the wallpaper. Or would it be a matter of coughing up silicone from the lungs, bringing me, as a patient had a few months back, large gobbets of phlegm in tissue paper, which she was sadly determined came directly from her implants by way of a bronchoprosthetic fistula."[1]

Or could it be an ear "hanging by a thread"? If so, I determined to be the soul of courtesy.

A pleasant, friendly voice introduced himself as an anesthesiologist at a pain clinic. He asked me if 11 years ago I had had a patient by the name of Mrs. Y.

So, it proved, I had.

"Well," he said, "she has come to me with bad headaches, which she has had for a long time."

---

[1] I almost want to say this would be impossible.

"I see," I said.

"I thought she might have sinusitis, so I took an x-ray."

I was certain that a "pregnant pause" followed, and I thought to myself again, "Oh, dear." She had apparently had some nasty facial fractures, nose, cheekbone, and so on. I wondered to myself if maybe her eye had now fallen into her nose, but the pleasant anesthesiologist went on, sounding just a little awkward, diffident, even a little embarrassed; clearly a sensitive person not wishing to be the bearer of bad news.

"The x-rays show what looks like a surgical needle that has been left in the back of her nasopharynx," he said flatly.

"You mean like a real needle?" I repeated inanely.

"I talked to our radiologist," he continued, "one of our best, and a fine Southern gentleman [a point I much appreciated, thinking immediately of all our own gentlemen radiologists!] and he has read it out as a 'metallic foreign body' but he called me to say that he would bet his life on it being a curved needle, like in surgery."

"Oh dear," I said for the tenth time, wringing my hands and making strange passes in the air.

We hung up. I fled to the lady's chart and carefully read the op report. It was not very illuminating. Nowhere in it did I read how I had forced a needle down her nose and buried it forever in her nasopharynx. I had seen her in the emergency room, where no one ever does a needle count, if indeed they are still capable of counting there at all.[2] She had an open fracture to her nose, fairly messy it looked like, with some flaps and so on torn up, and the nasal bones scattered here and there.

---

[2]This is not meant in the least as any sort of disparagement! Emergency room doctors, as anyone knows who has seen *E.R.*, deserve our utmost of sympathy and respect. On the other hand, by the end of a "shift," I do think there is quite possibly a diminution in their "counting" ability.

"My God," I now thought, "anything can happen, even probably winning the lottery without buying a ticket [as my wife and I sometimes think we just might]."

My thoughts tumbled one upon the other: How could I have lost a needle down her nose? What kind of hole had been in her nose? Could I have been trying to force a suture to go somewhere, putting my knees and shoulders into it, and broken off the needle without any remembrance? Had I had a petit mal seizure while sewing her up? Perhaps beneath the surface of my innocent, fluttery self there lurks a Mr. Hyde, and in some vile way I had become possessed that night long ago and, not dreaming of the evil of which I was capable, had forced a great needle down this poor lady's throat. Conceivably my family was in danger! Might I not be possessed to do the same on one of them, our dogs, our cat, or Spot, the little Guinea pig?

With an effort I shook myself back into reality. Never mind all that trivial business, I thought desperately, I've got to quick get some alibi, some decent excuse. True, the "incident" had occurred 11 years ago, but wasn't "discovery" the important word here? Would that not mean she would have two years now to contemplate bringing hideous action against me for "willful negligence with intent to harm, and for 11 years thereafter aggravated pain and suffering remediable only by torture in the courts, megacompensation, and punitive damages"? Between "now" and the trial I saw the needle, drawn by the Magnetic Power of The Law, burrowing ever more deeply into the nasopharyngeal tissues, moving irrevocably towards the cervical spine, into the brain itself to lodge in the very center of things, maybe even, "Ladies and Gentlemen of the jury," the Red Nucleus, thought to be the veritable seat of the Soul! Totally naked would I stand in court, melting down.

Having hung up the phone, I feverishly sought about the office, in my desk and under the wastebasket, for some harebrained explanation that my defense attorney, probably no "Dream-Team" for me, could render as distantly plausible.

Aha! It was she, it was she herself who put that needle in her very own nasopharynx. Yes, it was her fault! I saw as though by epiphany exactly what had happened. Yes, while I was absent after the surgery, dictating and writing prescriptions, she had inadvertently (key word that) coughed up some bloody phlegm, and either she or a helpful family member had grabbed a 4" x 4"[3] off the Mayo stand and given it to her to spit into. Caught up by its very teeny tip was the surgical needle, which as she threw the 4" x 4" to her mouth flung also the needle, which marvelously sailed posteriorly while the phlegm had gone otherwise into the 4" x 4" she held before her. The needle had been carried back by flawed fate, say a sharp intake of breath, where with its pointy point it had lodged in the back of her throat. There it had stayed, burrowing around for these past almost 12 years. It had nothing whatsoever to do with me.

"Case closed, your Honor."

In this wild tale I took solace and comfort.

And then . . . more epiphany! How clever the brain when forced by rude circumstance!

I called back the very pleasant gentleman anesthesiologist, whose number I had taken, and asked him in a very feeble, tiny little voice, scarcely capable of being heard, "if this lady had ever had any surgery in her throat before? Perhaps a little, teeny, weenie tonsillectomy?"

He had not taken any history to that effect but said he would discreetly find out.

He called me three days later to say he had talked to "my" patient and "yes [indeedy] she had had a tonsillectomy 27 years ago."

Christmas came after all and in just its good, old ordinarily hectic manner. Doctor X sent me a copy of the x-ray, and I saw immediately it was a great, big, huge needle that in my wildest dreams, even as Mr. Hyde, I would

[3]This is not a board, but a bit of gauze roughly 4 x 4 inches, used for sopping up a bit of blood, and on rare occasions I have even blown my nose with one, but it is much rougher than a Puff.

never have used. I had, of course, suggested that we get in touch with a fine otolaryngologist, and the pleasant anesthesiologist had arranged for "one of the nicest Southern gentlemen you would ever want to meet" to see her.

So it proved. The Southern gentleman of an Ear, Nose, and Throat specialist called me after he had peeked at her through the flexible nasopharyngoscope to say that he had located the needle, and that it was happily out, no harm done. It was the classic needle used in olden times for tying off nasty blood vessels in the tonsillar fossa. Apparently it had simply "popped off."

I learned that the otolaryngologist who had done the tonsillectomy has been dead for some years. He is in his own Heaven. He is just fine and his memory well honored in his profession. He is disencumbered of the telephone, beyond the pale of e-mail, and even subpoenas. My erstwhile patient is just fine too. Even though she is happy to have the needle removed, her headaches had nothing to do with its presence. The Southern gentlemen up in Georgia are treating her for a bit of sinusitis, and she is getting better.

I am happy too, even though I think I am a little more jumpy when the phone rings, but, as has been rightly said, I think by Kenneth Branagh, "All's well that ends well!"

Or could it have been "Much ado about nothing"?

ANCIEN RÉGIME
SYNDROME

We are being seriously guillotined in Tallahassee. Blood is running in the streets. Madame Defarge is knitting names. The Jacobins are at it. Our privileges, almost aristocratic in terms of the decades we have accepted them almost as "Rights," are being stripped from us. We are becoming *sans culottes* ourselves.

Well, let's hope I exaggerate, but something for sure is going on that is not very easy.

No, the guillotine is still (barely) in its closet. I do not hear tumbrels in the streets. Yet I think we are all capable of feeling just a dash more empathy for Marie Antoinette. Like us, the latter-day physician, she was used to her privileges. She could not help it, after all, if she happened to be Queen of France at the wrong time. Like ourselves, just perhaps, time and circumstance caught up with her, she was dealt a bad rap, and people of political rectitude unfairly heaped upon her the worst opprobrium. It is partly a matter of getting even, for us perhaps as for her, even if she never said that stuff about "let them eat cake."

She, like us, was actually a nice person, who adored her children and worked hard to support her image in a difficult court. The discomfort she had to put up with was more than any of us would impose upon our dogs and cats. She was not even allowed to relieve herself, really scarcely given a pot to pee in, if the moment was impropitious in terms of court etiquette and protocol. Like us, she had many demands heaped upon her. It was a pity she did not marry Mozart when, at age eight or so, he asked her.

When she was thrown into a filthy prison, to await execution, the contrast between her former exaltation and sudden degradation was, and remains, poignant: the stuff of classic tragedy. Whether we physicians are, as a whole, or just up here in little old Tallahassee, being rendered similarly tragic is a moot point. We may not be thrown in prison, but we are certainly being thrown somewhere, even conceivably o-u-t.

Some private practitioners, not already employed by an HMO, might disagree with my analysis. Accordingly do not consider these remarks anything more than a personal, rather jaundiced view. But as I perceive it, as succinctly as I can, business, I mean real Business, which has been chasing the medical profession for the last decade has, up here, caught us. We have been pounced upon. Even if we survive with our heads, will we be able to adjust?

The facts are that one of the larger HMOs in our area, indeed one formed as an IPA by a local excellence of physicians some 10 years or so ago, has decided under its new ownership that it is damn well going to cut care costs from some 91 cents on the dollars, to a more business-like ideal of 83 cents. Our local physicians' organization has spent much time and energy negotiating with the HMO on this and other matters, but suddenly . . . just like I suppose any business can decide to do if it pleases the board room . . . the HMO peremptorily broke off talks just when we thought we might be getting somewhere. Appearing on the table instead came a quite perfunctorily stated set of new propositions, which included the fact that costs would be cut, or we physicians would have to pay the overage out of our own pockets, and that, in order to control these costs, the HMO might even close its panel, decapitating who knows who of us.[1]

---

[1] As contrasted with being "capitated," by which is meant a method of paying a physician a lump sum for seeing as many patients as possible in the shortest period of time. Also, loss of the head, as in having it chopped off, an event devoutly to be avoided as well.

Our privileges, our autonomy, the *noblesse oblige* by which we have always practiced, and have been able to enjoy practicing, is, finally, seriously threatened. Like any group of aristocrats, we holler, consider it "unfair," and protest that the historically hallowed meaning of our role in society is being unconscionably ill-used. It is hard to believe that all this could be happening to us, who have been long trained and accustomed to the knowledge, tacit though it might have been, that ours has indeed been the aristocracy of the professions.

The Jacobins and the jackals are upon us. We are scattered here and there, everyone for himself. It is sad.

And what is happening in Tallahassee, as I write this, is that most all of us, to some degree, find ourselves bewildered and frightened, perhaps finally indeed "fodder" in the revolution under way in the "management" of health care. Never mind that this "management" is in large measure one of the greatest scams our nation has ever been treated to, besides which even the great silicone implant debacle, turning on a mere few billion dollars, pales by comparison. Never mind that it is little comfort to think of this revolution as something that inevitably should have occurred. After all, when you think of a trillion dollars (or whatever the figure) of "health care services" out there, surely it makes sense that real businessmen, real administrators, lawyers of course, assorted politicians, hangers on, the envious and all the rest should quite understandably wish to get a "cut" of this gold, Croesus-like in its quantity.

What has been required, and now has been discovered, was the means suitable to the need, as well as the creation of a proper jargon compatible with giving the movement its correct political "spin." "Cost containment" and other such chimeras and shibboleths have sufficed for the purpose, allowing the interjection of extraneous, financially interested parties into the former hallowed "doctor/patient" equation, siphoning off what is now there for the taking, and in the process (this I do not doubt) paradoxically adding its own enormous but uncalculated cost to the price of medical care. The establishment created to run us, I would guess, costs a good deal more than we ever "wasted" allowing patients to stay an extra day in the hospital.

The French revolution, and the Napoleonic wars that followed, cost France and Europe a great deal more in suffering and economic loss than anything the Ancien Régime ever spent on their cakes and dancing slippers. And how much, one wonders, is really achieved by such spasms beyond money and power being shifted from here to there? Those things we have so taken for granted for so many years with an almost aristocratic disdain (at least I think as perceived by some) are now being thrown back in our faces.

And it ain't cake.

I hope it proves at least mildly digestible cornbread.

Well, so far at least, unlike Marie Antoinette, society may yet claim to need us, so maybe we can keep our heads.

THE
HOMELY

INTRODUCTORY: THE HOMELY

In the homeliest of things and thoughts are the great differences often made. "For want of a nail . . . ," as they say, and so forth.

I think again of Anne Frank, who so dramatically validates the point. That an adolescent girl, who died alone and unknown, her dreams of some day making her mark as a writer brutally cut short, should have been in spite of those cruelest circumstances uplifted after all to that pantheon of writers best expressive of her times, and in her case perhaps the most revered of them all, is nothing less than the homeliest of miracles. That her diary, that most homely instrument of adolescent confession and hope, trampled afoot in the outrage of her abduction, should have yet survived to become the most poignant memoir of a world war, is in itself a paradigm for the extraordinary in all our lives. That she who was so fiercely victimized should have, out of such ashes, arisen as the "victor" over such callous cruelty is a latter-day proof of all possibility.

In one of the following essays, as I attempted to understand a little something of chaos theory, I found it rather hopeful, and helpful too, that out of such seemingly small things, iterating and reiterating upon themselves, what we are justified in calling miracles do occur. The flapping of that now famous pair of butterfly's wings in the Himalayas, causing a waft that has repercussions even to the extreme of a tornado half a globe away in Kansas, is now indeed cliché. We live in a world where none can say, but where that "least sparrow which falls" is remarked upon, and the universe made different.

In these homely details lies an essence. It is said that Napoleon lost the battle of Waterloo, "a near run thing" the Duke of Wellington called it, as a result of his hemorrhoids and not being able to seat his horse. What bit of health by the physician's intervention, be it ever so humble, might but result in some fulfillment scarcely to be imagined? What bit of action on the part of any of us does not result in the most profound repercussion? I myself, homely as it may be, have many times altered ever so slightly the overly aquiline line of a young lady's nose, and Lo!, it is as if she has been recreated, and finds herself with some remarkable new confidence. I have treated the most homely zits and seen as a result the most powerful transformations. All of this, of course, we all know; the point is homely in itself, and I forgive myself in its making only as a result of the pleasure I hereby take in expressing my perspective on it. I have noted before how delighted I am to have been given the opportunity.

And so follow these homely fragments, which I put into this category because, I assume, I could not quite fathom whether they tended towards matters "Good" or "Bad," acknowledging that for the most part we are all of us a little uncertain as we choose between this and that; for "Good" and "Bad" can often enough come strangely disguised, as do "Hot" and "Cold" when mixed in their infinite possible proportions to become something tepid.

As for "Homely," it is of course everywhere, amounting to the backdrop of the stage on which good and bad present their opportunities. Yet it is more than that, for there is nothing passive about "Homely" either, because in ways "curiouser and curiouser" it reaches out to grab the center of the stage.

Who knows when and who knows why? Perhaps quarks know, but they are not telling; and we are left to make our choice, and maybe that will make all the difference in the world, and the universe too! Perhaps we are those gods, as Conrad Aiken described it, "above a chessboard world," who possibly "utter words profound, and shake the star-strung firmament with a fateful sound." By our least choice and action.

REQUIEM FOR A "COOKIE"

In spite of Death, life prevails somewhere.

I do not know how many of you have ever grown a frog. But the "Grow-A-Frog" people of Three Rivers Amphibian, Inc., 668 Broadway, Massapequa, New York 11758, will be happy to supply you with the ingredients and recipes, all for only $12.95, shipping included.[1]

After placing your order, experience has now taught us, within two weeks, perhaps depending on the moon and the mama frog's inclinations, the Grow-A-Frog tadpole and complete kit will arrive. The impedimenta consist of a plastic cube with convenient hole in the lid, a fragment of artificial weed, and some pretty little pebbles appropriate to tadpole dimensions. A small spoon and a packet of tadpole food that looks exactly like Peter's 20-20-20 fertilizer are included. A delightful little booklet comes with this rig, containing pleasant drawings of many a happy frog, plus words of wisdom respecting both the external and, to remind you of Claude Bernard's[2] emphasis of this point, the "internal milieu" of your tadpole.

This young tad is no longer, I suppose, a true amphibian because one of its great granddaddies, deciding that the crime rate ashore was too high, withdrew to the atavistic deeps once more. Amphibian or not, his arrival sur-

---

[1] I do not speak for Three Rivers Amphibian and can well understand if the price of frogs may have escalated in the interim since we had ours.

[2] Famous French physiologist of the 19th century who studied and emphasized the delicate "environmental" balance obtaining between each of our internal organs and their functions.

rounds itself with a certain excitement. He (please use "she" here with equal emphasis at your discretion, because understandably I do not want to do any injustice to the distaff side) arrives in a Styrofoam cup, with "Living Material," "Rush," and "Handle with Care" stamped all over the place, just like any everyday kidney for transplant, piece of porcine skin, or (if you're up to using them) leech.[3]

After unlidding the cup and introducing yourself to your tadpole, you immediately notice that he is in all likelihood (1) floating on the surface, dead, or (2) in a posture called "head-down, tail-up" which means a happy tadpole indeed. You can readily remember the healthy position for tadpoles by simply noting it as being opposite to our own, which in health is "head-up, tail-down." In any case, having read the literature, you can start right off talking to and admiring your tadpole.

Because this delightful creature, even when a fully mature frog-prince, lives essentially in his little aquarium, quite under water, you do not have to worry about him growing up to hippity-hop about hearth and home, leaving, for example, muddy tracks across the pristine, white tablecloth of your wife's beautifully set dinner table. When fully grown he is perfectly content to simply practice his underwater strokes, exercise his stunning frog thighs, and spread prettily the webs of his feet so that small children and physicians can thus see the delightful miracle of his bony structures.

But there is more! What about the further miracle of God's handiwork as the tadpole loses his elegant tail and the four limb buds sprout forth, growing before your eyes until he becomes a veritable essence of Platonic Frogginess. Is this not, I beg you to acknowledge, a living lesson of ontogeny recapitulating phylogeny (or is it the other way around?) for the seven-year-old, as well as a happy little pet to call one's own?

---

[3]Making a comeback in medical practice, but will never reassert the popularity they enjoyed for blood-letting purposes that they possessed in their peak year, 1838, and which I predict will never offer frogs much competition in the marketplace of family pets.

"What would you like to name him?" we all asked Meredith, daughter of the aforementioned age.

"Cookie," she immediately responded. It seemed a highly attractive name for a tadpole. We all ate one (a cookie that is) with milk as we watched him, head-down and tail-up, gulping.

Perhaps the gentle-hearted reader should read no further. Alas, we are even now awaiting Cookie V. There is no need to give an elaborate clinico-pathological dissertation on the mortal illnesses of Cookies I through IV; suffice it to say that Cookie I died, we think, from an overdose of garlic essence introduced inadvertently into his immediate external milieu (never mind how that happened). Cookie II was DOA, and Cookie III died mysteriously a short time after his arrival. But such hopes we had for Cookie IV! He had been moved out of the kitchen to what we call rather pretentiously "The Library," because there is a book in the room and noth-ing very noxious like garlic going on. For two and a half weeks we clapped our hands with pleasure, watching his little limb buds grow, flaccid at first without their muscles, but at the end beginning to stroke feebly with the hind legs. He was a bright spirit indeed, flashing in his little aquarium, turning into a real frog. The morning of the day of his death he was all head-down, tail-up, yet gone by 2:00 P.M.

My wife called me at the office, and we all mourned. At dinner we went over the sad facts, reason struggling to know how one can be head-down, tail-up one moment and floating on the surface the next. We ultimately came to the conclusion that Cookie's fate had been sealed that very morn-ing by none other than myself. The final diagnosis was "Death by the acute onset of morbid obesity." Meredith, responsible child, had fed him his spoonlet of 20-20-20 in the morning unbeknownst to me, who untrustingly had then come dithering along to feed him yet another spoonlet, unaware that this would be a mortal draught. The instructions had, my wife reminded me gently, carefully emphasized that only one spoonlet should be given daily because something horrible, if not exactly acute obesity, would rapidly set in as a result of this sudden surfeit in whatever is his diet.

I called the "Grow-A-Frog" folks who are delightfully patient. At no expense to us, Cookie V is en route, but not without my feeling obliged to remark something or other about this greatest of mysteries, Life and Death.

Pretty bathetic (sic), one might hazard, but perhaps death in its more humble forms can be a little more easily thought of, and comforts thereby derived. I am not myself, as I think was ascribed to Schweitzer, particularly affected when I step on an ant. (I believe it was an ant that he hated stepping on.) I would suppose that in the scheme of things a tadpole is not much more marvelous than an ant, so it becomes clear to me that the death of Cookie has less to do with the death of Cookie than our perception and regard for Cookie's life. We had become familiar with his little gulpings, took delight in his head-down, tail-up position, and had examined his hind legs through a magnifying glass. As Conrad said about Lord Jim, he was, so to speak, "one of us." He had become translated into a value greater than mere dollars and cents and postage.

I worried a bit for Meredith's sake that the whole experience might turn her somehow callous, teaching a perception that death was capable of simple remedy by the dialing of a 1-800 number. I am glad to say that such has not transpired. Even though we did not have full funeral services for Cookie III or IV, our collective memory yet endows them with meaning. The lesson seems to be more one that in spite of death life remains, comes again, hope springing eternal even in the aquarium. Accordingly we shall, like Grant before Richmond, "fight it out on this line if it takes all summer," and I am fully prepared to keep having Cookies. My image is that whatever number it takes they are all worth it if we are to achieve a great white frog. With Cookie IV we came very close, were almost able to shake his foreleg so to speak, and so Cookie V may be the frog for us. Let us, I say to Meredith, carry on. Let us even rejoice, and think of Cookie indeed as a metaphor for ourselves, swimming about in this aquarium of a universe, gulping and metamorphosing, head-up or head-down, with hope in our hearts.

But take note, I might add, not to overindulge, particularly on tadpole food, and go easy on the garlic too.

A TOUCH
OF TOLERANCE

I recently found myself practicing my "style," my rough canvas hat à tête, in the hot tub of the Hotel Peabody, just off the I-4 Wonder-World in Orlando. Although I did what I shall call "a lap" in the double, Olympic-sized pool, it was a sufficiently intimidating experience so that I felt well content withdrawing to the more cozy security of this tub. With the water to my chin and my hat brim in its circumference almost touching its surface, I felt happy as a hippo and looking forward to dinner.

My torpor was suddenly arrested by the hauling into view of a pair of ankles, followed by knees, a couple of thighs, and clearly the rest of a lithesome feminine figure entering my nearby precinct, no one else being present. This is one of those difficult social circumstances: Do you remain quite still and quiet, or do you doff your cap and formally make an introduction? It seems a little rude, in a great hot tub, for two people to sit silently staring at each other, merely turning pink.

After the usual moment of mild confusion, I decided to turn up the leading edge of my canvas brim and address this very pretty, youngish lady with words suitable to the dignity of my years. She responded, and one thing leading to another I asked her what she was doing in Orlando.

"I'm taking a course," she replied, "for 22 weeks in how to be a chiropractic assistant."

"How delightful," I exclaimed, "to be spending 22 weeks in the Hotel Peabody taking a course! It seems a very pleasant way to receive an education."

"Oh, I only come one weekend a month, and then I get my certificate."

Now, as you are surely willing to grant, I am perfectly open to all manner of reasonably honest means of fending through life's mysterious waters, and feel no particular passion about "alternative" forms of medical treatment. Indeed, if it tends to do no greater harm than most other endeavors, e.g., driving automobiles, having a martini, practicing plastic surgery, I am content to leave well enough alone. Even so, and having little knowledge of chiropractic other than that my office is surrounded by theirs, along with pizza parlors and astrologers, I thought this might be a means of slyly getting some insight into the educational experience of the chiropractor or, if not himself, at least his assistant.

"How very interesting," I said in my blandest tone. "Do tell me what you are learning, for instance this weekend?"

I fear I tread on thin ice here, not wishing to do any particular curriculum an injustice, but the following was the exact answer given, which I thought interesting: "We are learning about bone pain."

"Oh," I said, "what is bone pain?"

The response was, "Bone pain is pain in the bone."

I marveled a little at the earnestness of her reply, coming as it did from a young lady who looked every bit as intelligent as Bo Derek, although she did not have those little braids.

I was driven to removal of my hat, actually exposing my pink skin to UVB. "Is that all there is to it?" I asked. "I would have thought there might be a little more to understand than simply that." But she could elaborate no further, and merely went on to describe in quite exhaustive detail how the entire day had been spent pounding home this homily regarding bone.

"Well, you certainly deserve a break in the hot tub after all that. But tell me," I continued, "what lecture have you enjoyed most on one of these weekends?" I assumed an avuncular tone.

She then described in some detail the weekend devoted to the "Soul," not only how the soul (as I think most of us would agree) plays an important role in the healing process, but lives forever. Being neither a cynic, skeptic, atheist, agnostic, nor perfervid fundamentalist, I shared with her that this seemed a belief worth believing by whatever glad means one might contrive. We had a merry chat about the soul. She told me in an almost conspiratorial whisper that she did not herself believe, in relationship to the soul's health, that people necessarily should have "an adjustment" every six weeks, like some chiropractors advocated; and she thought that such a matter should perhaps be left up to individual discretion, sometimes.

Having never had an adjustment of my bony self, nor I guess by implication a straightening of my soul therefrom, I was left without comment. Our conversation wound gently down into the more prosaic, with my agreeing with her that she must indeed have a wonderful "Boss." After some final desultory remarks about how people died in hot tubs, especially if they drank wine concurrently, I withdrew.

My wife and I conversed about this conversation at dinner. For what it is worth, we decided that the world is made up of a great mass of differing ways and means, and trapped within the limits of our narrow perspective, especially that of a hot tub's, we cannot properly weigh or discover the full meaning of any increment that makes up a part of the mess. (See "Hope Out of Chaos," in "Good.")

Whatever one may think of chiropractic, or Rolfing, or (gasp!) plastic surgery, in isolation their meaning may elude us, may appear trivial in fact, and be defined more by the prejudice of the perceiver than by what, whatever it is, that is perceived.

We concluded that one must be generous and kind about these things, if for no other reason than from an awareness that we too, as physicians, are "perceived." One cannot expect more generosity than one is prepared to give.

Not, of course, that we necessarily must include in this plea for our tolerance the PROs, IRS, HCFA, HMOs, DPR, or the color puce.

THE POWER NAP

I had the marvelous and rare experience the other day of taking a nap; not long, mind you, nothing at least long enough to be accused of simple sloth. In any case, often and tritely said, it was not the quantity but the superb quality.

For starters the surrounding atmospherics were delicious: children off someplace beating their brains out, wife sitting quietly in her comfortable chair dashing off some needlepoint, and I lying down to read a dash of George MacDonald Fraser. It started to rain. I heard it dripping from the eaves outside our bedroom window (the gutters, of course, have been clogged for months) and I thought of the Conrad Aiken poem about ". . . in the hanging gardens, there is rain, dripping from the eaves and bells of flowers . . ." and something about "drawing slow arpeggios over pools . . ." and some other stuff, and was, suddenly, deliciously asleep!

I woke up quite giddy with it all, but so delightfully refreshed that I determined that a holistic health principle should be premised on the nap as opposed to, for example, vertebral subluxation, zodiacal signs, low cholesterol diets, acupressure, moxibustion, football, or even (dare I say it?) jogging and other fatal forms of exercise.

It was quite revealed to me that The Nap is the answer to the world's individual and collective problems. In the fevered search for simple answers, what could be simpler? Why even trouble ourselves with "research," that slow accumulation of knowledge that simply leads to diphtheria vaccine, polio immunization, and the eradication of smallpox. A Big

Theory, well merchandised, is what we need. In The Nap we have a noninvasive technique for instant restoration, the only danger being the slight one of falling out of bed and hitting your noggin. With proper packaging, and the invention of a few words of wisdom from ancient Chinese philosophers of oriental napping techniques (never mind the Frenchmen's tryst *après-méridienne*), the package could surely be sold with great gain to the founder of this College of Nappery. It is simply a matter of presentation. If it can be done so profitably with something as abstruse as a subluxated vertebra, why not with The Nap, which lacks only being surrounded by a fabrication of technical jargon to give it modern credibility.

Remembering my earlier essay describing my meeting with the lady-in-training to be a chiropractic technician, my avid readers will note that I am still musing not only on chiropractic but the holistic practice of health care in general. As well, I have had an immediate experience of some curiosity to me relating, if not directly to chiropractic, at least to the more peripheral methodologies that orbit the mainstream of modern medical care.

A youngish man with a fine red beard and flip-flop sandals was referred to me. He had a biopsy-proven cancer on his back. He came with his good friend, an acupuncturist, in tow. It became quickly clear that although he could acknowledge the need for surgery, requiring conceivably my services, he wanted no part of anesthesia or any internally distributed medications which might unbalance his yin and yang. Well, I do respect peoples' attitudes, really.

Accordingly, after considerable bureaucratic hassle, I contrived to discover a hospital where I might remove the tumor using cold steel while the acupuncturist provided anesthesia by twirling a needle in the toe. My only provision was that we might have an anesthesiologist standing by "just in case" and that I might, "just in case," arm myself also with a touch of Xylocaine.

It was not easy to make the incision and, indeed, I only got about an inch. The patient gave what I suppose one might call a "whoop," and with his opinion reconsidered, we added a regimen of IV sedation and local anesthetic. The acupuncturist made some apologies to his friend, touched with a few explanations, and we were all very jolly together. Indeed I do not think my patient's experience rendered him any more skeptical about acupuncture (a friend is a friend in any case) but only that in this particular setting it didn't work. I think I thought, surrounded as we were by the aura of modern surgical and anesthetic paraphernalia, that perhaps the proper electrical ambiance was disturbed, rendering the acupuncture technique ineffective. It would have worked better, I believe, if we could have performed the surgery in maybe a dark but holy cave.

Well, as I noted in my last trenchant essay, *chacun à son goût*. Some people more than others are more keen to see life reduced to simple terms, and this is where chiropractic, acupuncture, and holistic medicine in general have an intrinsic appeal. As physicians with a long history of medical experience behind us, we are acutely aware that the great discoveries have been made only through the very slow accumulation of little blocks of information, hard won, but when gathered together at the right moment produce a sudden and marvelous blossom. The shamans of "alternate medicine" present us a blossom; but theirs has no stalk nor any root which, beginning darkly, produces over generations, cell by cell, the sturdy stem bearing bud and blossom. It took Leeuwenhoek, Spallanzani, Semmelweis, Holmes, Pasteur, and a long list of others to produce the revelations of Lister. I may be doing someone an injustice, but I cannot think of a single instance of basic discovery made by a practitioner of holistic medicine that has rendered the health of humanity more secure. In any case, how do their claims compare to Jenner's study of vaccination and the subsequent eradication of smallpox?

But Humbug will be forever with us, and in generosity perhaps we can allow that in it some will discover comfort. Let us hope as well that there will always be sufficient intelligence, such as that of this readership, who will contrive to keep such means and methods in proper perspective.

On the other hand, if you accidentally take a nap and awaken refreshed, revitalized, witty, gracious, and clear of thought, join my trend and take more seriously to snoozing. You could also for a mere $19.95 send for my pamphlet exclusives: "Power Napping," "How to Make a Million Dollars While Napping," "Great Historical Naps," "Bust Development Through Napping," "The Nap as a Corrective to Alopecia," "Enhancing Your Virility Through Napping," "Lowering Your Cholesterol By Napping," and "Napping with Your Cat."

Reading these are guaranteed to put you to sleep which, come to think of it, is not a bad idea, for the rain is again dripping from the eaves, the children are still off somewhere, and a great lassitude is sweeping over me. Maybe I will again wake up a charming figment of myself, my dull headache gone, my joints supple, and all my vertebrae well aligned.

"PRACTICING" MEDICINE III: RELIEF OF BOREDOM

I was charmed the other day to be invited by our local radiology group to a kind of soirée, the occasion being in honor (as the invitation announced) of "National Breast Awareness Month."

For starters, I had not been aware that "the breast" was quite so needful of a whole month to make ourselves aware of it. It seems to me it has awareness enough, particularly when you compare it to something like the pancreas, which can hurt a lot more, and only the most skillful can even speculate on where it is.

Nor, given my professional sensitivity, am I very sure I will attend this festivity because at the outset it has a suspicious ring. What are the radiologists up to? As everyone knows, they live for the most part in little rooms without windows and meet (even together amongst themselves) mostly in the dark. Can one really trust such penumbral types to come up with a wholesome view of our anatomical parts? I suspect that this whole invitation has merely to do with some new form of ray or magnetic field that they want to perpetrate upon us at probably great expense, using the breast as a guinea pig because it is such a handy organ with such slick media appeal. Of course I may be doing the radiologists a very serious injustice, and the party they are tossing may be the result of a most pure humanitarian motivation. Who am I, furthermore, to demur when someone comes along and indeed, even in print, tells me to be aware of breasts for a whole month?

To be fair this should be quite a good party, and I think I will indeed go if my wife will let me. The radiologists hereabouts are a rather fast crowd who drive around mostly in Porsches and Lotuses. I have always supposed that their confinement to such a shadowy world during the working day justified a few high jinks and fast moves when at their leisure. In any case, more power to them for finding ways to alleviate the boredom with which we all, after all, must day in and day out contend. So this party, introducing a whole month of breast awareness, seems to me a very happy and perhaps pace-setting initiative.

Of course one can overdo things, or even get into trouble when, in all innocence, one experiments with the relief of "boredom." I am reminded, for example, of that delightful neurosurgical case I read about a number of months ago. The setting was domestic, and clearly the gentleman's aspirations were well intended. It was only because of the merest little accident that they ended up by being not quite so well resolved.

This fellow had read somewhere about keeping "excitement" in marriage, and he laid a crafty if ambitious plan. Instead of coming home to watch the news, have dinner, and fall asleep on the sofa, he selected an evening when his wife would arrive shortly after himself, giving him time to put on his Batman costume. The article understandably could not dwell on the logistics of this operation, but when his wife came home she was tied, with a strong rope, to the bed. He then apparently climbed up onto the dresser, fully outfitted as Batman, to attempt a flying leap in order to "rescue" her from her trussed up plight. The *dénouement* was to include the ravishing pleasure of her falling in love with him as Batman, candlelight, wine, and strict romance. As so often happens when things are carefully calculated, the unexpected intervened: he slipped from the dresser striking his head, and fell bleeding and unconscious at the feet of his wife, leaving her screaming for the help of neighbors. They came in due course, and the remarkable curiosity of the scene was rather embarrassingly revealed. Batman recovered his senses with scarcely any help from the neurosurgeon, and just two or three little stitches from his good old family plastic surgeon.

The moral is that when the out-of-the-ordinary is attempted and goes awry, the sequelae will probably be much worse than when things simply go wrong from a routine habitually familiar.

So I hope the radiologists know what they're doing, and don't find themselves in more trouble than they bargained for.

On the other hand, if this comes off well, maybe other specialty groups could arrange something fun and festive for other organs about which we should be aware. The heart, of course, is the chief of these. In a sense the heart is a little irritating because we are so constantly being made aware of it, and already endowments are simply replete with money for it. I suppose the heart deserves this. When you get right down to it, however, it is nothing more than a rather stupid pump, even if it is such a good money raiser, and long ago captured St. Valentine's day.

There are many other more neglected organs deserving a month of "awareness." Indeed, I can rapidly enumerate more than the 11 left over after breast month is done with. I will be glad to hear from anyone interested in which organs they think would make for a good party. I myself am curiously partial to the spleen, an occult and mysterious, velvety-smooth bit of anatomy; I even think a good month for the bladder and prostate would be OK. Urologists usually are a happy-go-lucky, throw-a-nice-party bunch. Of course, forgive me, the skin deserves gentle April for its awareness month, and more plaudits than it usually gets because, contrary to the heart, it is a highly intelligent organ that keeps us looking good at parties, masterfully regulates our temperature, blushes and tans, and can grow a handsome mustache.

How about throwing a big picnic with martinis in the month of May for Batson's plexus?[1] And even a few cheers in June for the epididymis,[2] at least.

---

[1] A racemose ragbag of fragile veins rambling around at the base of the spinal cord, named after their discoverer naturally.

[2] From the Greek: *Epi* (on) and *Didymos* (twins) A rather wild bit of male anatomy defining that curious portion of those tubes that carry sperm from the testicular "twins" onwards, upwards (hopefully), and thus outwards, highly convoluted for some reason, and occasionally subject to infection, in which circumstance you are diagnosed as having "epididymitis" or, as my father called it when once afflicted, "that damned Greek."

LECTURE CIRCUIT

As I write this, I feel particularly aware of my homeliness. I am, after all, thoughtfully preparing a "lecture" I am to give to the Division of Plastic and Reconstructive Surgery at the University of Florida School of Medicine in Gainesville, two and a half or three hours down the road from Tallahassee, depending on whether you pause for junk food.

My greatest fear is that I will be nervous, borderline manic, or even find myself hopping about. I once gave a lecture to a whole bunch of pleasant but somewhat formidable-appearing ladies who were "Daughters of Something or Other" on the practice of colonial medicine, weaving this elaborate topic around the interesting attitudes and medical insights of Cotton Mather.[1] After lunch, and a rather abominable soup, which I did not get to dip my roll into, they chained me to a lectern with a little light and a microphone, and I delivered my address. Perhaps it was the soup, but for reasons I have never been able to understand I started having a whole mess of PVCs,[2] which rather interfered with my delivery. When I opened my mouth, instead of words emerging, out came PVCs, at first kind of slowly but ultimately arriving like quick balloons, to burst about in the room showering

---

[1]This early New England Puritan Divine (1663–1728), who I tend to think would make the strictest Victorian appear by contrast a full-blown Libertine, also wrote one of the earliest treatises on the treatment of disease in Colonial America.

[2]Premature Ventricular Contractions, that is to say that your heart, instead of going "lub-dub, lub-dub," etc., goes "lub-dubby-lub, Dub," to the great alarm of the neophyte heart-watcher and even the fully trained plastic surgeon.

the ladies, who looked grim about what was going on. They all had large purses, the kind you can whack a footpad over the head with, and I thought hopefully that surely one of them would have contained a defibrillator. I clung to the lectern, which seemed rather higher than it should have been, perhaps because my knees were also sagging, and wondered if my failing physiology would complete the talk. I finished Cotton Mather off in a flurry of ventricular eructations, and sat down cheered not only by the gracious applause of the ladies, but by the fact that I was alive. We all dusted ourselves off and I bid the Daughters of Whatever a gracious adieu.

So that is what I mean about getting "nervous." On the other hand if, as was forbidden me on the occasion above mentioned, I can actually hop around, I mean more or less from lectern to floor, floor to lectern, stage to audience, or even climb up on ladders, I do much better. The activity takes my mind off the fact that a lot of people are turning an image of me upside down as I pass through their optic lenses, to land on the back of their retinas, and then get translated into God knows what by their occipital cortex. But acrobatics when giving a learned lecture is frowned upon and, to tell the truth, I have never seen a debonair, experienced plastic surgeon, or any surgeon, or even anybody, get away with it. I need to project a composure suitable to what I shall call the "dignity" of my experience, homely though that may be.

It crosses my mind to grow a mustache, but to grow a mustache is something that would only cause my children to guffaw at me, and would take this business of lectureship too far. On the other hand, mustachioed though I won't be, I hope there will be a little desk (not a tall lectern) that I can kind of sit on (not at) at an oblique, casual angle. I want very much to give an impression of easy confidence, no matter how fabricated, enhanced by a kind of maturity of experience, enhanced further by the lightest *soupçon* of humor with of course a dash of wry wit sprinkled amidst a degree of scientific skepticism. Yes, that's it!

Actually, I suddenly have in mind Dr. Gilbert Snyder, Bravo of a plastic surgeon I always thought him to be, who talked to my group when I was a resident. Never mind his impeccably cut suit and the elegant length of his long legs, to which I cannot hope to aspire. I have never been able to get my inseam more than 30 inches, and at that sometimes stand on the posterior aspect of my cuffs. I cannot remember a thing Dr. Snyder said, except for something about an earthquake, or was it a volcano?, he once participated in. I will never forget the casual way in which he described it as "just a little earthquake" (or volcano), implying that he had either, or both, quite under his control. That's a real surgeon to me. That's what I want. That's the kind of imaging I am after.

Of course, I have to say something, too.

Like polyps for the proctologist, valves for the cardiologist, or *furunculosis impetuosa simplicans* for the dermatologist, the plastic surgeon enjoys talking about "flaps." These are fragments of skin and so on that are kind of lifted around surgically and allowed to wander on the body in hopes that they will plug some hole from which a patient's life-juices are outwardly pouring. The game plan, without which no lecture is fully complete in this specialty, is to talk about all the wonderful flaps you have done, demonstrating not only your superior technical skills, but ideally a tremendous amount of creative imagination, boldness, ingenuity, and the other 12 things that you learn to be when you are a Boy Scout. All these points, including that the flap lives at all, require demonstration by photographs taken from just the right angle with just the right lighting effects.

But because these matters do not compare with the breast or the heart's beating, I will not go into detail. Yet as a mere general application of a flap technique, suitable for the home, I should share with you my "Spanish Bayonet Folding Flap." Its application has probably saved some lives, and many eyes, as patients have approached my office. Down the narrow path to my front entrance, there is a seven-foot-tall Spanish Bayonet plant, which is about as subtle as an incoming Exocet. Its extremely sharp and tough points project

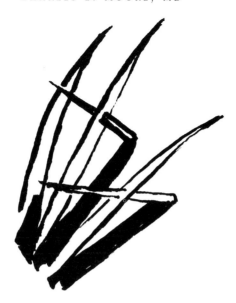

Spanish Bayonet Fold-Back Flap.

over the fence, and directly into the eyes of unwary passersby forging their way to my front door. I could, of course, slash the whole plant back, but many of my patients find it exciting *en passant*, and who am I, after all, to start hammering away at nature. So my (only slightly) invasive, non-mutilating technique essentially consists of bending one blade back on itself, and sticking its point through the blade a level higher, thereby thwarting the ambitions of this wicked hortus, which got its name by stabbing Spaniards through their armor. I would like to think this technique is original to myself, but frankly I doubt it, and so will not report it in our literature.

There is actually a lot more to lecture on. Come to think of it, I think I'll share with them the greatest scares I have ever had in my practice, short of delivering my lecture to the Daughters of Whatever. Also I must start polishing my shoes, for if I recall correctly Dr. Snyder presented to us not only his long legs but also a fine sock, ankle, and a lovely shoe. Perhaps no one will notice the tassel missing on one of mine, chewed off by our Christmas puppy.

I need also to check my inseams, of course.

DOCTOR–PATIENT–DOCTOR RELATIONSHIP

I n the last titbit I was taking my various pulses and clipping my toenails in *preparation for a lecture I was scheduled to give at the University of Florida* Great Teaching Hospital in Gainesville. This was at the invitation of Dr. Hal Bingham, Professor and Chief of the Division of Plastic and Reconstructive Surgery. Even though he is retired from the Professorial Chair of the Department of Surgery, under whose formidable aegis is organized the Division of Plastic Surgery, I was deathly afraid that the ghost of Dr. Edward R. Woodward would be present, and standing behind him naturally the ghost of Theodor Billroth II, and maybe Billroth I[1] also. These images daunted me somewhat, and as I scraped in my memory for fragments of homely cases and circumstances that have occurred in my practice, I wondered what I could possibly have to say to such distinguished pundits. Even the residents in training would have done a good deal more microvascular surgery than I, and I thought rather ruefully of how I must almost be shown which end of a microscope to look through. (It's the end that sticks up tallest.) I had hopes that

[1]Theodor Billroth, 1820–1894, one of surgery's greatest names, a surgeon who among many other German surgeons and physicians gave that country a leadership in the world of medical practice that it held until the ravages of the 1930s when, within a decade, the Nazis destroyed a tradition of excellence and, indeed, the honor of a profession. A great friend of Brahms, and accomplished himself at the piano, he is famous among surgeons for his bold and innovative techniques, still in use, which with right gay abandon swung loops of bowel hither and thither, hooking this with that, bypassing pathology here to connect with there, and of course including the time honored "Billroth I" and "II" procedures, affectionately known to every surgeon and medical student.

Dr. Hollis Caffee[2] would be there, with his delightful beard, and Dr. Leonard Furlow,[3] a scholarly gentleman if ever there was one, and from whom one can always take comfort, and learn an oodle as well.

But, remembering my terrible run of PVCs when I lectured on Cotton Mather to the "Daughters," I thought I had better go into some kind of training, or at least have a physical examination. I had not had one for a while, but because I have a great mess of life insurance on my head, being a consummate family man, complete with many dogs and cats as well as the usual adolescents, etc., it seemed to behoove discovery whether I was in sufficient good fashion to withstand the rigors of the lecture, hoping (a bit selfishly perhaps) to postpone any major transfer of monies from the insurance company to this wonderful menagerie surrounding me. To put it briefly, could my body stand another outbreak of PVCs?

So, and feeling rather proud of myself for doing it, I quite myself made an appointment to see my veritable physician. The last thing I wanted was to have a run of PVCs and ventricular fibrillations while lecturing to plastic surgeons because, clearly, I'd be a goner. They, of course, would all jump to their dermatomes and prepare for an emergency skin graft, but I am not sure that does much for heart stoppage.

My doctor, by the way, is Terry McCoy, MD, a lively figure of a fellow, known not only for his Irish affability but also as a rising star on the scene of local, state, national, and international medical politics. As a matter of fact, I think in the past he shook the hand of then President Bush who is said to have told Jim Baker that he thought Dr. McCoy a good shake. On the other hand, the President may have been confusing Terry with his wife, Toni,

---

[2]Dr. Caffee is now Professor and Chief of Plastic Surgery at the University of Florida, having assumed Dr. Bingham's mantle.
[3]Dr. Furlow, now retired, is famous for the charm of his wife, too, and also for his research on tendon healing (a tricky business that!) and for the invention of an ingenious method of repairing a cleft palate.

who is absolutely dynamite, and possessed of a lilting Irish idiom and manner that would make John Wayne give up Maureen O'Hara in a tinker's flash. (See "Working [a Little] for Food.")

I've had other doctors too: Jesse Judelle, MD, a delightful name locally and an astute physician indeed. But Jesse, with very great kindness and compassion, eased gently into that good night the passage of both my parents from this world to the next. Somehow or other I could scarcely bear that he should see me off too, for being reminded by him of all else I would simply have to burst into tears. When I go, I hope not to be blubbering, but with a kind of graceful charm about me, a dash of wry wit, my boots on, and perhaps a little mustache like Errol Flynn. Come to think of it, much of this description seems to me apropos to the manner I would like to assume when I give my lecture at the University of Florida.

In any event, Dr. McCoy seemed an apt choice for my needs. I think all too often people choose their physicians because of the colds they may need treated; whereas the true test comes at death's door. Would you be comfortable dying in the presence of just anyone? I should hope not. Get someone who, if you are too weak to project the right stuff and image yourself, will help you do it. This is why I've got Dr. McCoy. Who knows? Perhaps I could look forward to his wife coming to shake my hand in the process too, before I blink out.

I had my physical and I think I "passed," almost with flying colors. Of course, there's a little hypertension but, what the hell, it only takes three seconds to toss down a few Vasotecs each morning after brushing your teeth. An extremely creaky joint was noted; it is due to an old lacrosse injury, but I sometimes try to pass it off as being from a Zulu arrowhead in my hip socket, achieved in Matabeleland where I won the Victoria Cross defending the "station" against tremendous odds with the young Michael Caine. Of course *everyone's* cholesterol is rather high, but McCoy's treatment is to regard it with mostly a little Irish wit and charm.

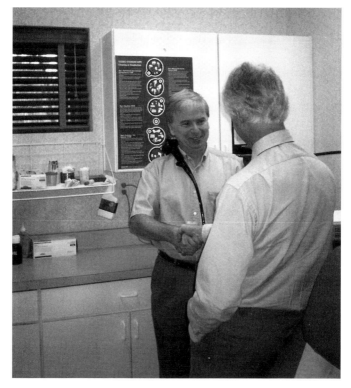

The author is congratulated by Dr. McCoy,
President-Elect of the Florida Medical Association, on his absence of polyps.

The part of the examination of greatest interest, invariably, was my sigmoidoscopy. It is what I believe is called the icing on the cake. The point here
is to maintain complete composure, forgetting none of the social graces, and
carry on without a hitch in the casual conversation you happen to be having
with the doctor prior to the *entré* of the examining tube. For practicing charm
in an awkward situation, this is a lot better than just walking about with a book
balanced on your head. We talked, I believe, about "the flowers that bloom in
spring," and the Zulu arrowhead in my hip. I gave only one almost impercep-
tible gasp when the tube poked my spleen (delightful organ!) and so passed
this test with flying colors. Although I got only a B on my physical exam, I got
an A in sigmoidoscopy, which averaged out pretty close to an A-. Dr. McCoy

says I may shortly be hearing from Alpha Omega Alpha,[4] an honorary organization I have always coveted belonging to, regarding an Emeritus Certificate.

In any case, deemed fit to give my lecture, I sallied forth to Gainesville accordingly, armed with a few slides, incunabula, and a bunch of hieroglyphics written on a 3" x 5" card. Everyone was perfectly delightful, shook my hand, and listened to me with what I shall describe as curious expressions on their faces. I ended up, interestingly, having far more to say than time to say it, so felt distraught and pressured. I told them about the scariest things that had ever happened to me in my practice, and everyone congratulated me on not having been sued silly. Dr. Bingham fed me a light lunch, and it was a great pleasure to see him, whom I much respect.

Then I went home, proud of myself for having had absolutely no PVCs during my talk. I wonder what it was about the Daughters of Whatever that gave me such a fearful attack of them? They really were, believe me, a very nice bunch of ladies.

---

[4] A prestigious society to which only the most brilliant medical students are elected. After I got an A in our very first anatomy test in my first semester of medical school . . . for which test I studied inordinately in order to contradict the received opinion of many that I would most likely flunk out quickly (I not only believed them but was acutely aware that I knew no German) . . . I entertained brief hopes for myself. It all came, however, to naught, and I graduated (at least) as a more or less "gentleman-scholar," but by no means AOA.

STENDHAL SYNDROME AND OTHER ITALIAN SYMPTOMS: I

The other evening, while needling and forking about in the mouth of a poor fellow brought to the emergency room with a nasty laceration, half cutting off his tongue, I inadvertently rammed the needle (he had inconveniently lept for the chandelier) through my left index finger. You have already read how much I enjoy doing this. I cursed loudly *sotto voce*, and after the uncouth fashion of our modern circumstance, required by all the cultural and physiological implications attendant on such accidents, the nurses ran around drawing blood from the patient for HIV testing.

"Oh well," I thought to myself, "at least I did not come down with Stendhal syndrome." For those not familiar with the treatment of this condition, or conceivably even its diagnosis, it is a morbid affliction peculiar (if not invariably) to mostly travelers to Italy of a particularly sensitive, artistic, and, I might say, on the whole rather intelligent type. Maybe, come to think of it, I should have come down with it—but I get quite ahead of my story.

My tale, and such non-observations as I have to make on the practice of medicine and surgery in Italy, begins in the halcyon summer of 1990. Among the debris orbiting my desk, there surfaced an envelope of foreign texture and address. Its origin, indeed, was a street the name of which reminded me remarkably of a spaghetti dish I once had at the Casa Vecchia, a posh South Florida pizza parlor. It did not feel like an envelope full of spaghetti, and I comforted myself knowing that at least it could not be a bill, because I have not bought any Lamborghinis lately. Accordingly, I boldly slit the envelope with my beautiful Italian letter opener (or is it an English fruit knife?) and withdrew the contents. The letter, in English happily, was from Doctor and Professor Umberto Veronesi announcing the "First International Conference of the European Society of Mastology," hereafter known as EUSOMA, a new organization, sprung fully armed, or at least already with an acronym, from the head of Professor Veronesi.

He described the organization's purpose as being to study and disseminate information on the epidemiology, diagnosis, treatment, and everything else in the world that can be thought about breast cancer. The goal was that those in all specialties dealing with this disease should meet across the board, discuss, share, collate, disseminate, drink, eat, and stand around, and that somehow or other I could even come too. It was to be held, good grief Charlie Brown, in Venice, in some wonderful, ancient structure on the *Isola di San Giorgio*, a mere five-minute *vaporetto* jaunt from downtown St. Mark's Square.

My pupils dilated, and in impeccable Italian I said, "*Wow!*"

In a twinkling, I considered how (dignified though my years have become) I have never been anywhere international for anything medical, although I know Disney World, Amelia Island, The Diplomat, and The Fontainbleau pretty well, and have even been to New Orleans. I have never seen what real European doctors look like, and I was particularly keen on what sort of feathers plastic surgeons wore over there. Then, somewhat more slyly, I thought how I could take this opportunity to sneak my wife along to Venice (being careful to leave the children home) and write a mess of it off on my tax return. In my excitement, I suppressed the clear knowledge that no matter what I have ever "written off" on that nasty return, I have never received any money back from the IRS, and my taxes have never gone down.

In due course, skipping over some bureaucratic stuff and other confusions in my faxed exchanges with Professor Veronesi, I gave my Visa number, which knows no language barrier, and became a smart new member of

EUSOMA, thus permitting me to go to the meeting absolutely free. My wife and I fluffed up our passports.

Then came Desert Storm and rumors that Sylvester Stallone and one of our better symphony orchestras had canceled trips to Europe for fear of terrorism. My interpretation of this uncharacteristic show of timidity was that Rocky I–VI, Rambo I–?, and an entire symphony orchestra were clearly much more "high visibility" targets than us chickens, and that we could probably sneak through the terrorist net. Furthermore, we thought it might be pleasant to see a bit of Italy without Sylvester Stallone or even any particular background music. So over we flew indeed with almost an entire jumbo jet to ourselves, permitting us to stretch out fully on the seats to sleep after drinking all the extra champagne left over from the absence of Stallone and the orchestra. This was heady stuff for a small-town solo practitioner, but I want you to know that I remained calm and steady, bearing in mind the high standards of the AMA and whoever is its present president.

We stayed in Rome only a couple of nights, and my only observation of medical practice there was to note a beautiful brass plaque around the corner adjacent to our little hotel. It was mounted beside a baroque entrance discreetly announcing the office of a plastic surgeon, whose hours were from 5 to 7 P.M. "Now that," I thought, "is real *virtu et dignitas*." Such hours any of us might aspire to: cultured, elegant, etc. But it was the simple plaque itself I took as an example to heart. If only Florida would allow such discretion, in no way surrounded by neon signs or billboards depicting the Venus di Milo and other assorted bosoms.

We had shopping to do before setting off for Venice. I had an ache in my fourth lumbar vertebra, and wondered if this might be an early symptom (artistic temperament that I am) of Stendhal's disease. Apprehension in this case was quickly eclipsed by the prospect of the adventures that lay ahead; not to forget, of course, the *panini* loaded with fresh everything:

pale shades of pink prosciutto and balsamic vinaigrette; olives and cheese; a lovely wine *al fresco* beneath the azure sky of an Italian Spring; and gazing at my wife with a highly subtle and suggestive eye while chomping into my succulent *panini*.

Marcello Mastroianni could not have done it better.

Read on for the thrilling conclusion.

STENDHAL SYNDROME AND OTHER ITALIAN SYMPTOMS: II

The day before yesterday, as I was descending upon
Florence from the high ridges of the Apennines, my
heart was leaping wildly within me . . .

STENDHAL

As we caromed down the high road to Florence, my heart was leaping wildly within me. This, I thought, is merely the result of a flush of adrenalin stimulated in my manly soul by fast driving in real Italian traffic. Aside from my leaping heart, I felt as well ever so slightly vaporous and a little brittle: the early signs, possibly, of Stendhal syndrome.

At least I took encouragement from recalling how well my sensitive spirit had dealt with Venice, that most romantic of cities, with my nerve endings succumbing to only an occasional quiver. In Venice had resided the ostensible purpose of our jaunt: The First International Conference of the European Society of Mastology (EUSOMA), an organization intended to draw together in harmonious colloquy varieties of medical specialists having at least a remote interest in the study and treatment of carcinoma of the breast.

"Oh, clever," I thought, "is he who creates a new organization by holding its first meeting in Venice!"

Had Dr. Veronesi announced that this inauguration was to have been in Oshkosh B'Gosh, I fear I would have politely excused myself and simply carried on, but Venice, oh watery dream, oh poetry, oh city of gilded domes and shimmering lagoons, of dark canals, and beautiful ladies with mysterious eyelashes, of old men with perfect manners, oh Ruskin, oh Byron, and, as my yawning travel agent suggested, "How about Thomas Mann?" He had seen the movie.

Having arrived, we dragged our luggage and a huge bouquet of flowers all over the place, pausing for refreshment and directions in St. Mark's Square. I was prepared for the pigeons. Prior to our departure from Tallahassee, I had in secret practiced (as well as my four lines of Dante) the line I now got to deliver while flushing out half a dozen or so from beneath our little table: *"I piccioni sono sfrontati."* The novice linguist loves to flaunt his phrases, as you know, reaping the reward of getting to tell those who don't particularly give a damn what it all means. In this case I proudly announced that it meant "the pigeons are cheeky." They were too. As my wife rather more pertinently pointed out, they were courting by the thousands, half of them males with their feathers fluffed out and walking in circles with stiff knees, and the other half ladies with their feathers beautifully flat and coifed, paying no attention whatsoever. We saw no actual acts of passion by these *sfrontati piccioni* but, of course, did not wish to appear too curiously rude in a foreign country. We preferred, as we had been trained by our travel agent, to simply let the idyll that is Venice permeate every fiber of our very being, as well as two bottles of a light red regional with dinner.

The next morning, shaking off only the mildest headache (not an early symptom of Stendhal syndrome), I presented myself in my best shoes at the vaparetto stop near St. Mark's Square along with a large gaggle of European-looking ladies and gentlemen. There were a few English, who still contrive to surround themselves with the light-hearted insouciance of Empire; more or less rational looking (of course) French; some stolid German lady and gentleman doctors who might also have been discus throwers; a lot of Italians speaking only English; and a large mass of eastern European types that I got mixed up regarding. I sort of stayed to myself, the "mysterious loner," humming a little tune from "The Third Man," starring Orson Wells and Joseph Cotten.

On *Isola di San Giorgio*, we all gathered in what seemed to be a beautiful church, nothing whatsoever like "Meeting Room A" at The Americana in Bal Harbour. I found myself between a Romanian on my left and a Yugoslav on my right. I now know that I should probably have introduced myself as Charlie Moore from Tallahassee, but felt constrained, mostly I think by the very large jaws and premaxillae of both these gentlemen. I took a little professional pride, as a plastic surgeon, in recognizing their mandibles as clearly tracing back to the famous "Hapsburg Jaw,"[1] and the rest of their bones as tracing from the Schwarzenegger gene pool. Because I know no Romanian or Croat, and in Italian feel only comfortable with the word "*sfrontati*," I simply hunkered down and attempted to make my bones look a little larger.

Then came some general lectures and other stimuli, wherefrom I learned that breast cancer was most statistically prevalent in New Zealand and least in Guatemala (*nota*: Research the prophylactic attributes of the maize kernel in this disease) after which the main colloquium broke up. I went to the room where all the European plastic surgeons were hanging out, and listened to them give papers remarkably like those I hear at Disney World and Bal Harbour. Having by now achieved the gist of the conference, the day being lovely and luncheon *al fresco* with my wife beckoning, I discreetly excused myself from the meeting. We were just barely able to afford window shopping and a few remarks to the pigeons in St. Mark's Square, took a power nap, and later dined elegantly at the Gritti Palace Hotel. There we had the entire dining room and staff to ourselves, because everyone else, including Stallone and the orchestra, were busy watching CNN reporting from the rooftops of Baghdad. By contrast, I took some pride in practicing old-world manners on my wife, who is beautiful and necessarily long suffering.

Now we were barreling into Florence, my pupils dilated and my heart beating like Stendhal's. I made a mental note to send Dr. Frank Skilling,

---

[1]An interesting skeletal feature of the Hapsburg clan.

ophthalmologist and one of our enlightened local *literati*, a postcard *molto sfrontati* for having suggested to me that, being middle-aged and vaporous, I was a prime candidate for Stendhal syndrome.

He had told me of an actual case with which he had been involved: a lady of sensitive intelligence referred to him by a local neurologist with signs and symptoms suggestive of neurological disorder, perhaps an episode of frank or incipient cerebral ischemia. She had always been a lady of studious predisposition inclining toward the romantic. She had read Benedetto Croce and Cellini; she knew all about Lorenzo the Magnificent and Piero di Cosimo; she had read James and knew Vasari; she knew the birth date of Michelangelo and could even spell Pollaiuolo. The whole gorgeous retinue of the Renaissance paraded about in her brain, in the clear outlines of a Uccello painting, complete with all the horses, banners, and spears. She was middle-aged, I think a spinster, and had saved carefully for this artistic pilgrimage. Alas, upon arrival in Florence she shortly thereafter had palpatory feelings, some arrhythmias, PVCs, and lightness of the head, tinglings and curious weaknesses of the limbs and syncopal diatheses. She consulted an Italian physician with a discreet brass plaque who, fearing the worst, advised her to return immediately to Tallahassee. She did, in deep distress that her journey was thus cut so rudely short. She saw a neurologist and also Frank, but by then her symptoms had abated and her eye grounds were quite intact. None could make anything of it until Frank brilliantly diagnosed Stendhal syndrome.

For this sensitive, intelligent soul to arrive in Florence, her whole being in this case aware of its magnificent cultural past, is it not to be understood that the experience was overpowering? Where to start? What to see? How to see it all, and time so short? The syndrome is one of cultural and sensory overload, inability to assimilate so much that is so palpably and suddenly at hand. Once the dreaded symptoms strike, you must be simply flown home forthwith!

Well, suffice it that I did not succumb: too tough and insensitive. My wife and I had cleverly decided to see very little except what stumbled upon us, and instead ate spaghetti and *panini*, that magnificent Italian Renaissance version of the hoagie, slathered in oil and stuffed with superb complexions of prosciutto. Oh, not to worry! We galloped through the Uffizi, gaped at the Botticellis, and adored the Bronzinos, and I got a pain in my back as any sightseer must, but I knew, perhaps a little ruefully, that it was not Stendhal syndrome! It was from carrying lots of luggage.

When we finally got out of the Uffizi, we had a glass of wine, seating ourselves comfortably at an outdoor café, the sky azure above. We walked across the Ponte Vecchio, glancing at the shops full of golden trinkets, and ascended the hill to our high hotel in an ancient tower mentioned touchingly by Elizabeth Barrett Browning. My wife pointed out to me the small violets growing out of a weathered wall. In the warm sun their bright faces leapt, as it were, heavenward, and seeing that homely sight we wondered at how marvelous it all was indeed, every smallest leaf!

And what a fine dinner we had, and wine yet again, and I was not, yippee-yi-yo, flown home to my neurologist!

POLONIUS RESURRECTED

A nd remember," sez I, "to thine own self be true and don't dress too foppish or French and," fluffing out all my greying feathers so as to appear impressively round, "don't forget either Luther's 95 Theses, the Golden Rule, Millard's Principles, Pascal's Pensées, the Hippocratic Oath, and, for God's sake, don't cut too close or long some scholarly surgeon's sutures at Shands!"[1] I hopped up and down and flapped my short wings, adding with a knowing cock to the head, "nor never ever stand behind an arras with your feet sticking out from under lest some fool with a rapier mistake you for mayhap the King of Denmark."

Thus have I been having a marvelous time fluffing myself up, casually tossing off "Great Truths" and other *bon mots* in the direction of (extraordinary delight) a neophyte physician who I fancy has even lent a graceful ear.

Indeed, speaking of Ms. Pike's ears, they are prettily turned (plastic surgeons look at superficial protrusions for which on behalf of us all I beg your indulgence), neither outstanding nor too in, with a neatly defined anthelix[2]

---

[1] Shands Teaching Hospital, synonymous essentially with the University of Florida Medical School, Gainesville.

[2] The little ridge within the outer rim (helix) of the ear, missing when ears are "outstanding," which is to say sticking out, or more colloquially "Dumbo ears." Many sensitive children, teased unbearably, are driven to surgery for correction; whereas others, contriving to live happily in symbiotic balance with their ears, go on to become great movie stars (Clark Gable) or Princes (Charles). In Japan, curiously, largish ears that stick out are positively equated with intelligence, and for all I know people there may pay plastic surgeons to make them do so all the more.

and a scapha[3] of lovely proportions. Now, alas, she was about to leave us for Rosencrantz and Guildenstern–land in Gainesville to learn of pie in the sky at Shands Teaching Hospital and become in due course a fine physician. My feathers sagged and my inseam shortened (see "Lecture Circuit") as I thought of her lost within the depths of Shands' mighty mazy corridors. On whom now could I rend the air with hot homilies? On whom now, as she neatly cut my sutures to perfect length, could I glance with telling innuendo, rendering my eyes steely blue and making the pupils big and little as circumstance suggested?

For I have had in my attendance, indeed in my part-time employ these summer months, an actual medical student; nay more, a lady medical student, and at that one of neat intelligence, sweet disposition, kindly temperament, and expressions of interest and curiosity regarding what I do, which have fallen most happily on my, sticking neither in nor out, ears.

Now mind you, I don't mean to suggest that I do not enormously appreciate my small staff, who honor me with their friendship and courtesy. But with one's staff, as you know, one simply must plod a wearier path, the day in and day out of being handed by them wicked pink slips to return sundry calls, to bring piles of charts that you already thought you had dictated, and otherwise heap your desk with all manner of artifacts and old bones. They, in their turn, are subjected to my whimperings and wringings of the hands, sighs, groans, curses, and a fierce tantrum once when, over almost nothing, absolutely everyone in my office burst into tears and thought it was all my fault.

Samantha, the above-mentioned Ms. Pike, is otherwise. Although she knows anatomy and biochemistry, she came unburdened by theses and eponyms, a young lady quite at home with her own ideals and purposes, modestly and gracefully expressed. Skipping the hyperboles, such grace is in itself worth preserving and highly sufficient.

---

[3]Boat-shaped; that nice flat space between the helical rim and the anthelix.

I mention these points, so delightfully a part of Samantha's character, not only as happy truth, but also in relation to a conversation briefly held while my wife and I were dining out recently with two attorneys and their wives. The remark was made by one of the lawyers to the effect that it was a pity that "doctors lost all their humanity in medical school." Never fear, you can be assured I followed that up with something pretty snippy about how lawyers lost all their honesty. But excusing the jaded remarks of my quite honorable legal friend, I took advantage of the opportunity to consider more acutely their perceptions in the light of Samantha's forthcoming medical school experience. Surely medical school does not make us less humane! Horrified, I gave Samantha a copy of a Trollope novel as a talisman against this threat, and snuck in to boot mighty words of humane wisdom over an occasional bag of potato chips.

For this I forgive myself, asking you to remember you are dealing here with someone who for 20 years has practiced in a kind of consummate isolation with no one to vent upon. We cannot, after all, ply platitudes on our peers who have learned their own the hard way. But Samantha was another matter; she was worth it, and I was paying her a salary anyway.

All summer she has remained in apprenticeship, and I have taken her through warts and moles, lumps, bumps, and how horrible is scar tissue. I have regaled her on all those points that the lawyers think are extracted from the neophyte physician in medical school. I have had her look at old tomes, and have shown her how to put in stitches. While waiting for a red light as we walked up to the hospital, I told her how being good in the practice of medicine is probably a more worthwhile ideal than being "perfect," the latter being impossible, and who can define it anyway. Of course I threw in, only by implication, "know thyself" and "honor thy profession" and "respect thy colleagues" and "you can't know everything" and "in our ignorance a little compassion goes a long way" and "whenever you feel afraid whistle a happy tune."

So these and other things I got to say, in right homely fashion, to a delightful and attentive young lady to whom I pay my compliments. I wish for her the very best and, I might add, consider that whatever she brings to our profession will prove a happy, humane credit to ourselves.

As for those lawyers, well, I suppose there are some honest ones. Would I, after all, be dining with them otherwise?

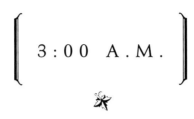

3:00 A.M.

I awoke about 3:00 A.M., having been startled into consciousness by a dream encounter (no need for details even if I could remember them) with Kim Basinger. Leap to conclusions if you like, but let me add my distinct recollection that in the final moments of the affair I was steadfast. In essence I told Ms. Basinger, "No, certainly not!" and to the stirring sounds of something like "Hail Britannia," with pink clouds and *putti* drifting about, I turned away to cast an adoring eye on my wife who was "off scene," shopping. Surely it is understandable to even a fairly phlegmatic temperament why such a dream would shock any red-blooded, young, handsome, rich, and charming male into quick disbelief, never minding mere arousal.

Over coffee with my veritable wife the next morning, I proudly informed her of my fidelity, even *in statu somnambularis* (?), and that if one can resist Kim Basinger in a dream anything is possible when alert and on the *qui vive*. I even confessed as well how it pleased me to think that I was staying with the times. Usually when I fantasize at a red light or in the dentist's chair, it is about some starlet of the '40s or '50s, or even of quite platonic relationships with people like, for heaven's sake, Joan Fontaine, whose crooked smile always intrigued me. But Kim Basinger, more or less as she appeared in "My Stepmother Is an Alien," her hair blowing outward by an electric fan unseen just within the bathroom doorway, is not fuddy-duddy class. My wife, of course, was very proud of me, and as I dutifully brought her another cup of coffee we took pleasure in thinking I was so neatly in her hip pocket, so to speak.

What I didn't tell her was that after I awoke my thought process was all downhill from Basinger. I suppose this is what Scott Fitzgerald meant when he wrote about it being "always darkest at 4:00 A.M.," Zelda snoring off an alcoholic binge at his side, and not even the *Florida Medical Association Journal* interested in publishing his work. In any case, I started thinking of all the people who could potentially sue me, and might decide to do so, faithful husband though I am. This train of thought invariably leads to further morbid concerns regarding lumps and bumps I have given people in the immediate past that they might not have bargained on, and which I can only hope will settle out with "time." My invariable response to the concerns of my bumpy-lumpy patients is to fall more or less to my knees and show them the whites of my eyes. Then I say, "Oh, give it some time," for the healing process after all takes a good year and frequently 20.

In this dark 3:00 A.M. instance I particularly thought of a lady who has some scars, compliments of my scalpel but no fault of mine, surely, which seem remarkably presumptuous, refractory, and in a phase a little too hypertrophic.[1] How long, I queried myself, can I keep her in dark sunglasses and a phantom operatic mask before she gets put off? I shall have to be, I say to myself, quite smooth and patient, show my concern and not allow any perspiration to flood my upper lip when I see her. She loves her dogs, and doubtless I will talk a great deal of "dog" to her and can maybe work "cows" up later on, for she has a herd of these also. But why, oh why, must she be the wife of a powerful figure up in Georgia from an area from which I have never had many patients, and had high hopes I might through her garnish a couple more?

---

[1] Overgrown, or blown, as in "hyper," and "trophic," as in a "trophy," e.g., the reward you get in the form of a permanent scar, being forever a memento of your surgeon's scalpel or some more nasty trauma. A hypertrophic thickening of a healing wound is very common, usually abating in the absence of any treatment, but on certain unpredictable occasions doing quite otherwise, to become ever thicker and heavier, itchier and uglier, and maybe even what is called a keloid.

This gloomy train of thought finally exhausted, I went on to economics in general. Forgive me for being the age I am, and for having been in practice for as long as I have, without having my economic situation fully in hand. I was sold (etc.) these terrible "tax shelters" just before the tax law of 1986 (surely no more need be said), and only lately my "trusted" insurance agent was indicted for having embezzled $300,000 not all of it my money but enough to discourage even me from keeping him on as my agent. Many people had warned me about him but, of course, I thought he was a nice guy. Now I am being importuned by insurance people once again, all of whom come equipped with the most magnificent policies ever made by man or woman, with favorable clauses beyond belief through companies all of which are rated quadruple A, four star, and two thumbs up by movie and other reviewers. Oh well, this too will work out.

Now it is almost time to arise and meet the day. I fall into a deep sleep for two refreshing, innocent minutes; then it's up to feed and put out the dogs and feed and let in the cats and, voilà, your devil-may-care-surgeon is ready to face the day with polished wit and tongue.

I wonder what percentage of people, particularly physicians, go through this 3:00 A.M. business. No one ever speaks of it, so secret is that moment. The shrinks, of course, say it is this sort of thing that keeps one sane during the day when you really rather need to be, but as for *serious* 3:00 A.M. anguish I think it deserves the utmost respect. I think of good physicians who are being sued unfairly and tried indeed by fire, of people struggling against demons, drugs, and real infidelities, of our patients who are sick, frightened, and in pain, or whose children are. I think even of the lady with the scars around her eyes, or the bump, for whom this means much, and who must think what thoughts at 3:00 A.M. herself, and of me to boot. And yet, for the vast majority, at 3:00 P.M. when we see them in our clinics, they are composed, understanding, patient, and revealing the best that people are. As a profession we are uniquely in a position to know and praise the restraints and courage that ordinary people, our patients, reveal to us every day.

Otherwise, now that you are awake (or have you fallen asleep?), I strongly recommend that you see *My Stepmother Is an Alien*. My wife loved it almost as much as *Cannibal Women in the Avocado Jungle of Death*, and maybe you ladies might even have an interesting dream about the co-star, Dan Aykroyd.

EVEN MOZART COULDN'T PURR

O ur dear old cat is dead, like Mozart, of kidney failure. *Unlike Mozart, he could not play the piano, but he often* sat on the keys slightly north of middle C purring loudly while I tried to more or less play around him. Vagabond, as well, had an easy dying and a lovely burial surrounded by adoring family, all of which Mozart was sadly denied. (I am not even sure if Mozart's wife, Constanze, made the funeral, and even the grave was a "common" one, unmarked, and lost forever.)

If at his going Mozart left us "The Magic Flute," Vagabond left behind in our memories the most remarkable purr I have ever heard, and none of us will ever forget it. It was the kind of sound that could act as a superb lubricant in the production of the "Music of the Spheres," which I picture as a bunch of very shiny ball bearings naturally needing a little greasing if they are to produce the kind of universal harmony for which they are famous. Vagabond's purr had a kind of universal quality, a form of sound with, yes, platonic ideality. Our eight-year-old daughter had the privilege of hearing his last purr as he lay but a bag of bones and fur on the floor of her room. He had spent the night there, and when she awoke she petted him; in his habitual fashion he immediately purred his gratitude and contentment and attempted to rise, arch his back, and respond. He could not, and two hours later he was found by my wife. Gone!

We had expected his death for a number of months and were amazed he "hung on" so long. We watched him carefully as he became more and more

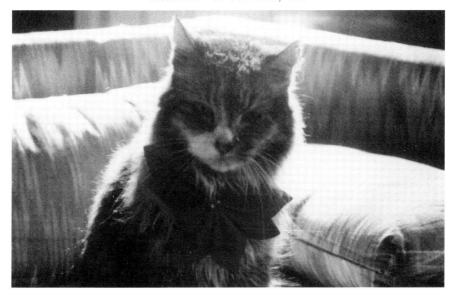

Vagabond, a noble cat, ?–August 21, 1991

emaciated, intending to "put him down" if we saw any signs of pain or discomfort. There were none, Bright's disease being forgiving in that respect, I think, and so he died a quiet and natural death, perhaps a blessing for cats in this world as well as people. Prepared though we all were, we were likewise astonished at the way his death tenderly affected us. Then, of course, in the best tradition of Kübler-Ross, other moods set in: "Kill all the dogs," I wanted to say, "what right have they?" I looked at Bunter, a great black Bouvier with a very thick skull, and thought of Hamlet's musings: "So excellent a cat that was, to this, Hyperion to a Satyr." Happily a kinder philosophy intervened, and never minding the dogs, we took comfort in remembering all this little cat had meant to us and would continue to mean.

My wife dug a deep hole in the garden, and I went to the nursery to bear home a stately red maple. We lowered Vagabond into his grave, wrapped in a fresh towel, and our eight-year-old made a pillow of flowers and scattered more upon his body. We planted the tree above him, to our eyes a happy monument to his memory.

From the foregoing, it is rather obvious that I have been thinking lately of "death and dying." Until I was 55, like most teenagers I thought I was immortal. Shortly after that birthday and coincident with my father's death, rather like Vagabond's in his being spared the terrible rituals of nursing homes and intensive care units, I was struck by the fact that no one of a previous generation now stood between me and eternity. Although I am mercifully unafflicted by any sorts of hypochondriasis, I felt twangs in both my hip joints sufficient to suggest that things wear out and turn to dust. As a matter of fact, I am driven to the conclusion that I really don't want to die at all, and have, in fact, some grave doubts about how I will ultimately face that reality.

Of course the PR people employed by Death glibly state that it is all "perfectly natural." Well, I don't think it's very "natural" at all. Getting up in the morning is pretty natural, and making coffee, and going off to work, and breathing, and conceivably watching a little TV, but death? I simply don't die very often, nor does anyone else I know except those extraordinary people who are "brought back" by a highfalutin medical technology. But even if you've had that experience it doesn't seem to me one you would want to make a natural "habit" of. I think I would almost, but maybe not quite, even prefer to watch a game show on television. In any case, to all those people who find death perfectly "natural," and go around blandly trying to convince me of the fact, I say let them have it, with their various apertures occupied by tubes and some ghastly poison being dripped into their veins. Then, despite all that, you are plucked away anyway and end up God knows where, for eternity. And even if you go to heaven, I'm not sure I would call that very "natural" either, because I don't think angels make coffee in the morning; they simply swoop around in their bed clothes, scarcely, I think, even getting to breathe. In any case, death is a ticket to no one knows where, but for sure it's not to the Dolphin Hotel in Orlando, and the vastness of that unknown rather intimidates me.

Well, so what? People, after all, have been whimpering about this state of affairs since time immemorial when the first hominids looked at the night sky to wonder what all the twinkling was about. So, to tell you the truth, I would like my going to be as Vagabond's, gently and with a purr. I would be complimented if anyone would regard my life in retrospect as I regard his: one of grace and beauty, true to himself, loving and loyal, courageous, and with the eye of Hyperion, commanding the respect of brute dogs who gave him wide berth, and whose presence near us seemed always a compliment.

Nor shall I ever forget (for sentiment's sake certainly) his mews of happy greeting on those hot summer nights, as I was returning from the emergency room at 3:00 A.M., when he would rush to greet me down the path to our front door.

We hope our children will be just like him. Even though none of us, not even Mozart, could ever purr as well.

ELEVATION
OF EYEBROW

The other day while idly perusing pictures of chromosomes, I was struck by the pure pulchritude of the X. It was such a marvel of size, utterly dominating the other 45, and rendering diminutive the poor Y, which bravely stood alongside.

Before you jump to conclusions regarding my attitude, I want you to know that I am a tremendous admirer of the great X, as will be demonstrably shown *vide infra*. Nor am I being sly when I say that when you have two Xs, voilà, you have a thoroughly marvelous half of the human species. It is this double X that stands for grace, elegance, beauty of form, the hope of virtue, and, yes, an extraordinary intelligence without which the Y chromosome left alone would very likely scarcely brush its teeth.

But beyond my credentials as a chromosomal morphologist who can recognize at any cocktail party, with its characteristic Q band, a double X person, the credentials permitting me to write hereon are exceptional in that (as you remember) I have been to Washington. Moreover I arrived at the very height of the Clarence Thomas inquisition, which you may somewhat recall.

Of course, I tried to avoid watching any of this *spectaculum spectaculorum* on television, concentrating my energies on my own lobbying efforts for the poor little silicone implant. But given the nature of the proceedings, and with television sets so ubiquitous and everywhere turned on, you could not escape.

Also, I was only three blocks from the actual scene, now famous, where a motley variety of distinguished Senators were pondering by due process whether or not Judge Thomas, based on his sexual harassment (SH) credentials, would be a good Supreme Court judge. I prepared myself to be ever so guarded and alert for incipient signs of SH in myself, and in the event happily have not embarrassed myself except once, when a lady with 180 pounds of XX chromosome stepped on my toe in the elevator with her high heel, causing me to groan suggestively. She took it, however, in good humor: She apologized and, of course, I apologized that my toe had been there, wanting to be sure that she knew I had not purposefully put it under her heel as some sort of veiled insinuation that I might be eager for worse or more.

But let me not stray from pure science.

As Descartes taught us, we must first seek the unassailable premise, the fact upon which all else will unravel. In this case can we deny that the basic principle must relate, after all, to the fact that there really is a difference between the sexes? But, as pointed out earlier, it is not only that the X chromosome is a Great Bigness, but also can it be denied that we gentlemen, no matter how hard we may try, will forever be missing one fourth of an X, turning us into brute Ys? Thus attenuated, the male of the species is clearly pretty well compelled to do anything he can to make up for the difference.

The consequences, as I think psychiatry corroborates, start in infanthood, when the male, understandably unaware that he is missing a quarter of a chromosome, discovers on the other hand that he has a curious addendum between his legs which little girls don't. He is often obliged, perhaps falsely, to transcend his chromosomal insufficiency by fluffing this masculine apparatus, and by the time he learns about the missing quarter of a chromosome it is sometimes too late to change an occasionally rude pattern of habit or thought.

In any case, having granted that there is a difference between the sexes, our task is to decide how we can live within these circumstances that seem so basic and enduring. I deign dreadfully to suggest that this can be done only by tolerating the difference, if not the rudeness, rather than trying to stamp it out like the unisexists of the far left, and James Thurber on the right, who wrote a short story titled "Is Sex Necessary?"

Flying back from Washington, I resolved to stand forth for a strongly intermediate position, committing myself anew to the arduous task of simply enjoying once again the XX–XY differential. I am not suggesting that male surgeons in the operating room wear swords and codpieces, nor plumes in their chapeaux, nor clank around in armor, nor that female nurses need to cinch in their waists like Scarlett O'Hara in the prequel, nor wear half a dozen petticoats in the Florida heat and humidity. On the other hand, there is (isn't there?) an enduring meaningful romance about such images.

In any case, even though we men are missing a hunk of chromosomal information, many of us manage to resist harassing ladies, and some even finally arrive at the status of being described as "real Southern gentlemen."

I do not think our greatest experts such as Senate Subcommittees, Geraldo, and Rosie whoever-she-is could define sexual harassment absolutely. When Rhett swept Scarlett into his arms after Atlanta burned, was that sexual harassment? What about that most interesting circumstance relating to Professor Richard Hummel of the University of Toronto who has been banned from the University swimming pool as a result of charges that he stared too hard at a lady and "repeatedly . . . swam beside her wearing a snorkel and goggles." I confess that I, myself, noticing the long, black eyelashes of a lady-nurse anesthetist interestingly situated above her surgical mask, once subtly wiggled my ears at her and lifted my eyebrows up and down real fast.

If you ladies think my explanations for these shenanigans are pale and jejune, and that missing chromosomal material is no excuse, I suggest that it is hard to understand what you are missing when you have never known it, and that's why men, trying to make up for the inadequacy, become famous chefs, Michelangelo, and (some) even surgeons.

In any case, without major genetic engineering and grim sociological change, I don't think men are going to change much from what they have always been, and I am not sure I think they should either. Someone is always going to offend someone, and I hope that we of the attenuated chromosome will not have to go around dreading intimidation if we comment on the length of a lady's eyelashes. Conceivably, there may yet remain a place in our relationships for a touch of (even) lusty humor, and I hope of innocent error.

Ergo, in summary, I say (with Descartes, surely) *vive la différence* but, believe me, I am going to work even harder around the watercooler (there is one in our OR) and elsewhere to treat all ladies forever after as a real southern gentleman should.

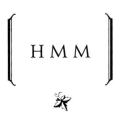

HMM

One of the physician's greatest prerogatives resides in the indulgence granted him in the use of "hmm." Considering that this expression contains no vowel and only two consonants, it is replete with a rich blend of association, as well as a unique ability to exorcise, explain, and encourage. Name two other consonants that do so much for your patients. That we physicians remain its master is a fact from which we may take comfort and, to some small extent, exult. The government, in any case, has not yet intervened to take our hmming from us, but that does not mean we should not be careful on this point and mind (to toss in a couple more consonants) our Ps and Qs.

The history and full exegesis of this happy term, which requires so much training to use wisely and well, must necessarily begin by consideration of "the Economic Questions" surrounding it, for it is here, as you will rush to allow, that the crux of the matter may ultimately lie. In the piously expressed, but possibly putative interest of cost containment, our hmming, the means by which some of our best diagnoses are made, may be disallowed and even removed from the *Manual of Relative Values*.[1]

But take hope! Even as I worry the point, hmm, if not the more fulsome hmmm, in subtle form may yet be retained in the CPT codes.[2] We are, after all, paid by an enormously complex system requiring lots of decimal points

[1] A system by which can be calculated fees allowable as charges to patients for various treatments, which if you do not do it properly can result in your being sent, at least, to prison.
[2] More of the same, i.e., of Footnote 1 above.

that only our office cryptanalyst can hope to decipher. This system of coding derives from the brilliant work of the so-called "Bletchley Group" which, by cracking the German code in 1940, allowed us on a scale of relative values to win World War II rather more quickly. The ingenious and hard-won principles that emerged out of "Project Omega" are now put to use by our office managers, who can brilliantly do it all in their heads. In my office my cipher-section even has quite a good time sending various cryptograms back and forth to Medicare from which finally emerges either an outright denial or a check for $3.78.

But let us move from economic questions to other reasons for mirth. Foremost among these is the fact that lawyers are not allowed to hmm at all. Each client is acutely aware that he is being charged 15 cents a second, with a stopwatch going, and that every time the attorney hmms it costs $10, both in person and on the telephone, depending upon the length of the hmm. On the other hand, let us fairly note, their relative value scale is much simpler than ours, constituted as it is by the simple expedient of suing everyone for no less than $2 million, and taking half.

But I am again distracted from my point, which is meant to be far more meditative.

The *Index Medicus*[3] gives reference to no prior articles on the age-old diagnosis of hmm; yet, through etymological analysis, we can clearly relate this term to a pre–Indo-European archetypal sound, ubiquitous amongst our hominid ancestors. In the pre-Ur and trans-Indus cultures, tossing in the Fertile Crescent, hmm relates closely to the earlier MMM root. The expression was, however, a blind alley linguistically speaking, which took language nowhere, though it has remained extant and meaningful particularly for physicians. The addition, on the other hand, of the vowels "u" or "o" to the

---

[3] The bibliography through which may be discovered articles pertaining to anything whatsoever that has been published of a medical nature, including even in foreign languages that no one can possibly read.

mmm sound gave us, clearly, "Mum" (*Lingua Britannica*) and "Mom" (*L. Amer-icana*). Mind, in any case, that when you hmm at your patient you are harken-ing back to the most remote antiquity of language, descriptive indeed more of feeling than meaning. The hominid protophysician *felt* things (as in itching) more often than he/she/it *meant* them (as in syllogistic solipsistic thought).

Our first historical reference to hmm comes from the great Ur tablet. It was discovered just prior to the Gulf War of 1827 when Saddam Hussein's great-great-great-grandfather was digging trenches prior to the "Great-great-great-grandmother of All Wars" against some small tribe. In this important tablet, which appears to be a bill for services rendered, it is clear that the physician felt no hesitation whatsoever in charging by the hmm. There are some 23 hmmings, which added up to the equivalent of one small ox, a she-ass, and (precise translation here has offered many difficulties) what appears to be a ticket to some early form of a football game.

Of course, we no longer charge such outrageous fees for hmming because it is now considered "low tech," and the government only pays, paradoxically, for more expensive, "high-tech" words and devices. Even so, hmm lives. It may come as a surprise, but even plastic surgeons hmm. My own use of it, of course, could not compare to that of the psychiatrist who spends his entire 50-minute hour hmming, but because I do at least half as much psychiatry as I do plastic surgery I am well acquainted with its semantic power.

My most vivid, and I might add grateful, personal full-feathered usage of this happy noise occurred recently when I was confronted by a lady who wanted me to remove the radio receiver her neurosurgeon had implanted into her brain. She considered its presence a perfidious plot on her sur-geon's part. For five years she had been, zombie-like, under his command, and made to do all sorts of things against her will. She broadcast to me at great length, and I hmmed away right merrily. When we finally wound down and my last hmm was hummed, I suggested that I was a plastic sur-geon, and really didn't know where the brain was at all. Hazarding one final hmm, I tentatively suggested that if she would return to the neurosurgeon, and explain her discomfiture to him in nice terms, he might take it out for absolutely free. Or, as an option, we could get a psychiatrist to locate it for us because he/she knows where the pons[4] is and the hypophysis[5] and enjoys all that kind of menial work anyway. She was highly gratified with this advice, and we gladly made her an appointment. She left thoroughly pleased not only with my acumen but my hmming. After her departure I sat down and let out one of the longest hmms I have ever attempted, and popped a whole bag of popcorn, that I instantly ate, washed down with a stiff Diet Coke, straight up and full of caffeine.

So there you have it. It is in such simplicities that medicine yet remains so subtle and marvelous. Surely, say I, "they" will at worst never be able to take that away from us! Ours is and shall remain the Long Tradition, reaching back into the mists of prehistory: the subtlety, yet also the simplicity, of what we can sometimes achieve with so little, not to mention the glorious satisfaction, after all is said and done, of sitting in our very own office regarding all about us as good, and eating our very own bag of popcorn.

It's enough to make one hmm, and with a contentment pleasant enough so that it even comes close to a prr.

---

[4]A most ancient bit of brain, just north I think of the medulla, responsible for all sorts of basic functions and perhaps some mischief too.
[5]The good old pituitary gland, I think, highly supportive of endocrinologists.

PANNICULAR-
LAPAROSCOPIC
SYNDROMES

I live a professional life that reminds me somewhat of the well-known phantom of the opera. I perceive myself, despite my Class V[1] liability status, as dwelling somewhere in the basement of the great Opera House of Medicine, every now and then making a wild-eyed, half-masked, half-asked appearance on stage, vaguely distraught, and hmming away not necessarily in the correct key. This is one of the reasons I am not very effective on committees.

Perhaps all of us, including even heart surgeons, work pretty much out of our own half-subterranean circumstance even though, like the phantom, we are necessarily acutely conscious of the stomping and howling on stage. I almost never see anyone else performing surgery or actually practicing medicine, except sometimes the emergency room physicians when I am called there. I am not even altogether sure what they do, never having seen the television program, although I enormously admire whatever it is. As an aside relating to continuing medical education, I think each of us should spend one week of each year with some practitioner outside of our own specialty in

---

[1]High Class, if you can so regard it, but who really wants it? After all, the designation sadly has nothing to do with how classy you might be as a surgeon or person, but only with the degree of risk your liability insurance carrier considers you to be as you practice within a higher or lower risk specialty. I think dermatologists and metaphysicians are Class I, paying tiny little premiums more or less, whereas neurosurgeons and obstetricians (Class VI) can just barely be considered self-employed, but rather instead employees of (a) the government and (b) their insurance company. This is one of the reasons why brain surgery, having babies, or having your wart removed by a plastic surgeon costs so much.

order to learn something of the tunes he/she hmms, acquainting ourselves thereby with a few of the phantoms with which he or she must contend.

Coming from what seems an ever-narrowing perspective, as I perceive my own to be, the practice of modern medicine strikes me as quite marvelous when I have the occasional opportunity to observe the breadth and depth of its application outside my own field. I would like to note accordingly the pleasure and interest I recently took in actually getting to work with other live surgeons, complimenting them in passing. More specifically I would like to identify a hitherto undescribed set of syndromes, the defining characteristic of which is the postmodern combination of fat with any other more classical need requiring surgery, such as having one's tubes tied, and particularly surgery utilizing that marvelous device, the laparoscope.

Sadly, I have not yet found any very happily valid need to incorporate the laparoscope into my own practice. But who knows? Maybe in due course the dermatologic and plastic surgeon can discover some means of introducing a skinny variance of this excellent device beneath the skin, and thus go tunneling about looking for creepies and crawlies. For some time, I am now ashamed to say, I actually wondered how laparoscopic surgeons were able to do all the marvels they did. I never understood how you could look through a 1½-inch tube, get your hand down in it armed with scissors and forceps, along with the scrub nurse's finger to retract, plus the pathology you were taking out, and see anything at all. My training, clearly, was in the days before the video monitor.

Now, as a result of recent experience, I know better, and so scorn the ignorance of my former self. Keen enthusiast that I have now become, I want a laparoscope of my very own to take home to fool with and fix, for example, the leaky plumbing in our downstairs bathroom. Using wonderful instruments and big video magnification, I would never again have to break my back wedged between the bath tub, the trash can, and the commode.

But, alas, the laparoscope remains peripheral to both my experience and my need, and I feel relegated to the sidelines as a mere envious bystander. On the other hand, I have myself discovered, and can now note to name by eponym no less, the following Syndromes of Laparoscopy and Fatty Symbiosis (SLFSes).

The first of these presented itself as a patient with Snyder-Zorn syndrome, a combination of gallstones and what we plastic surgeons blithely call "disproportionate abdominal fat" (DAF). Although gallstones and fat are not infrequently seen in common, along with the other hallmarks of "fair," "forty," and maybe even "a touch of flatulence," it is rare that treatment comprehends both gallstones and fat. At least in my experience I had never before been called upon in collaboration with the choledochocystic[2] surgeon to remove fat concurrently. In this instance, I had the great pleasure of hmming with astonishment as Drs. Snyder and Zorn deftly extracted the gallbladder through the laparoscope. While I awaited my turn at the fat, I watched the video screen, and noted perhaps three drops of blood being lost. It was all done with such finesse and exquisite delicacy in handling the tissues that it was enough to make me, as a plastic surgeon trained to respect that sort of technique, weep with envy.

Oafish enough I felt when the cholecystectomy was deftly completed, and I proceeded to my own brutal battering at the subcutaneous fat, applying to that rugged task all the finesse of a lumberjack sawing a cord of wood. I tried to put a good face upon it, and gasping for breath looked up at Dr. Snyder with a weak and sweaty smile and said, "It's rather like playing the cello, you know," a remark he accepted only in silence and the suppressed flicker of a

[2]That is to say "the gall bladder," a bit of anatomy to which no lobby I have ever heard of would want to devote a month to the appreciation of. It is an organ interesting only to those who are in pain because of it, or the general surgeon who gets to remove it. Its removal through a "Band-Aid" incision is one of the triumphs of recent surgery, and for this reason if no other let us honor it.

smirk. He left to drink coffee with his merry general surgeon comrades in the lounge, and once again there I was, alone, pounding away at lipocytes.[3]

Then there is the Dewey syndrome, a curious combination of what looked to me like feathers in the knee joint, and disproportionate fat elsewhere. As I humbly waited my turn in the operating room, much enjoying the charm and erudition of Dr. Dewey's discourse on the location of the knee and envying, as well, his easy rapport with all about him, I could not help but admire orthopaedic technology brought to such a degree of perfection. Once again the laparoscope revealed all, and the "roto-rooter" plucked out all those feathers, in a trice making the patient an outstanding tennis player. Dr. Dewey and his team were too busy to watch me do my suctioning, for which I felt supremely grateful, not wishing to be perceived by them as a mere half-blind, brute panniculectomist.[4] When I finished I was actually sweating and panting (a dainty plastic surgeon!) and they (brute orthopods!) were coolly discussing the fine points of the ligamentum cruciae.[5]

Of course the most common fat syndrome is that which comes in combination with problems related to the womb and associated other tubes and follicles. The removal of the womb, or a little cauterization of some tube, presents for many afflicted with this syndrome an ideal opportunity to come away from the surgery a size or two smaller, allowing a lady (necessarily in this case because it is well known that men do not possess wombs) not only to improve her tennis game, but to be able to tuck her shirt into

---

[3]Fat cells, known also as adipocytes, now famous for being in the wrong place.

[4]I must look up whatever is a "pannicule." I think it is a kind of off-the-wall, abstruse synonym for a fat cell, or (as has been already pointed out) a "lipocyte," which I think I would pronounce (particularly at a Class V dinner party at, for example, a Park Avenue address) with a short "i," as in ĭ. On the other hand, there are some who would fight over the point; and, paradoxically, when it comes to pronouncing "liposuction" I insist on the long "i," and am thoroughly offended by the short.

[5]Which holds your knee together, thank goodness!

her slacks.[6] Some of you may not realize that this is a quality of life issue, never minding your tennis score.

Understandably, I am eager to laparoscope something on my very own, and wish I could come up with some clever application. Meanwhile, I must fix the leak in our downstairs bathroom, and need to find a massive wrench.

I wish Drs. Snyder, Zorn, and Dewey had a sideline in plumbing.

[6]I apologize that this remark appears within what could be construed a facetious context. It is a homely detail, this being able to tuck in decently one's shirt tail, but of real and sensitive meaning to those who cannot. I have seen a strong woman weep with the pleasure of being able, once again, to do so following a judicious removal of her lower abdominal lipocytes.

THE BREATH
OF DEATH

I had an uncomfortable experience a few months ago.
A patient on whom two years prior I had done a facelift (the kind of
surgery that many beautiful but aging stars have "not" had) presented
herself in my office with a complaint. Childless, divorced, overworked,
and singularly hostile in her gaze, she pointed to her neck and demonstrated,
rather to my horror, a thick mass of scar tissue beneath the skin.

It measured about 4 x 4 cm, not quite visible but easily palpable, hard,
and tight. I made some fluttering passes with my fingers, and (not wishing
to commit myself) uttered a feeble "Hmm."

She replied to this . . . from her point of view not very helpful noise . . .
by saying, "Do you remember the plastic surgeon who was shot and killed
out West a few months ago?" Without allowing me a moment to say, "Oh,
yes, of course I do, awfully sad, had children, good man, remarkable case,
facelift too, wasn't it? . . . ," she continued: "That's what I want to do to you."

She looked at me, venom pouring pretty blackly from out her pupils into
my own, by now pretty well-dilated. I wondered if I should grab my flak
vest and put on a helmet. I wished I had handy my magic wand, which I
would have touched to my head, causing a "Poof" and my disappearance in
a small residuum of smoke. But my flak vest was at home, where I tend to
keep it because that's where the kids are; and although I am working on a
magic wand I have not got it perfected; at least I am not sure I can "come
back" once I have gone "Poof." So I kept a close eye on her purse and spent
the next 50 minutes, while my waiting room filled to overflowing-out-into-

the-street, talking with her, cajoling, listening, daring a wee bit of harangue, and finally parting. As we terminated our consultation, she seemed a tiny bit better, and indeed gave me a tiny little "hug." I kind of wondered if it was the tiny "hug of death."

I tried to tell her I did not understand what the big lump of scar was; that I had never seen anything like it so long after such surgery as she had had. Meanwhile I felt uncomfortably confident she might have very nearly meant what she said about wanting to kill me, and it crossed my mind for a few days to walk about with a white sheet over my head, and my eyes closed so she wouldn't see me. But in time I forgot all about it, and heard nothing from her.

In this interim I have, in rather more abstract fashion, given some thought to being murdered as an occupational hazard of the physician.

Might this not, in an anxious high-tech age, become a more popular option? For the present, however, I am not very aware of how many physicians are slaughtered in the line of duty. How many do you know? The first one I ever heard about was a plastic surgeon in Spain, who did some kind of penile implant on a young man. Shortly thereafter the patient marched into the plastic surgeon's office (was the implant not long enough? broad? or what?), and drilled him dead. Since then to my knowledge there has been the tragic murder of the aforementioned plastic surgeon in the Northwest, whose patient found that her facelift did not sufficiently render her "happy." It seems to me also that I read in *Medical Economics* about a doctor in Jacksonville who had his office shot up, and a few people I think injured, when a patient of his attempted to kill him off.

Accordingly, thinking I would actually do some research (!), I called the University of Alabama Medical School's 800 consultation number and finally was led to Dr. Tim Colson, who is in charge of the Occupational Disease and Hazards epidemiology section. I asked him if he knew of any articles about the murder of physicians by patients, because I was interested in not being murdered by one.

I put it rather blithely, telling him that I was particularly curious as to whether or not there were certain medical specialists more prone to being murdered than others. For example, I suggested, it seemed to me that plastic surgeons might be very prone to being murdered because we come across as a slightly breezy, dilettantish bunch and, therefore, irritating. As well, we are prone to perpetrating upon our patients little bumps and lumps that, coming unexpectedly, cause them to want to murder us right off.

But our category of risk is not nearly that of those who perform abortions, or even psychiatrists. I don't understand how any of them survive at all! Also on the highish side of this spectrum of risk I should put, astonishingly when you think how humble they are (despite the fact that you cannot get an appointment with one for months), the dermatologists. I can fully understand how a person with an intractable itch, unrelieved by cortisone, coal tar, and more obscure unguents, might simply take it out on his or her skin specialist.

In a lower category of risk, if not the lowest, I would guess might be the cardiologists and gerontologists whose patients, the blood just barely trickling through their muscles, are simply too weak to pull even a trigger, and certainly would be incapable of the kind of blow that would take the point of a dagger, bouncing off a rib, deeply into the heart.

Last, in the very lowest category of risk (oh happy they, who in the legal-liability category are so high!) are the anesthesiologists. Their patients certainly cannot kill them, because these patients are almost dead anyway, and even though thus "moribund" are yet tied down on a table with numerous straps, not to mention tubes, probes, esophageal thises and thats, plus that clothespin that anesthesiologists invariably now put on a finger in order to be sure that their patients have just barely enough oxygen.

In any case, hoping to verify my premonitions, I spoke with Dr. Colson and he kindly did some research in some kind of computer. He came up with curiously little, but sent me what he had. All of it had to do with mostly other occupational hazards, with no mention almost whatsoever of physicians, who perhaps are now so expendable that we are not thought worth the research. But it seems to me this area needs at least a little study, because after all we need a baseline starting *now* so that by the year 2001 we can note the patterns, write an article, and, of course, go see the movie again with the Strauss soundtrack.

As something of an aside, I would even go further and suggest that the names of the doctors thus murdered in the line of conscientious practice may deserve tribute, even maybe a bit of a small monument, names carved on it and so forth; but please don't put it in Washington!

In any case, you might be interested to know how my non-murder turned out.

It happened, in due course, that I ran into a family-practice type doctor in the hospital, passing her with a particularly chirpy "good morning." This ritual completed, she brought herself up, and turning asked to have a word with me. "By the way," she said, "do you remember Mrs. X, the lady with a purple ray that comes out of her pupils?"

"Of course," I said, "I know her quite well. I could not miss her from your description."

"Well, I saw her, and she has a classic case of scleroderma. It is all in her arms, with thick areas of contracting scar, the muscles tight, and probably systemic symptoms if not signs as well."

I was amazed. Scleroderma! It had never crossed my mind. I had been absolutely certain that the scar tissue in her neck, in some incredible manner, was all my fault, even without the aid of silicone.

I confess that from my own point of view it was a great relief to have understanding and a diagnosis.

But there is a great deal more to it than my own feelings. Never mind how it came about, but Mrs. X called my office, asking if I would do a "blood test" on her to find out what was wrong. I explained gently that I knew nothing of what blood test was necessary, but that it was more complex than just a blood count and potassium level. I told her I would accordingly call a rheumatologist, and having done so set up the tests, and made her an appointment to see him. The matter was complicated by her absolute refusal to pay anyone, lab or person, anything. The rheumatologist kindly saw her anyway, talked with her and gave her the benefit of his advice and what help could be offered. But sadly hers was a galloping, "malignant" process. She called me just recently, and we had a long telephone conversation. She described how she was taking leave from work and planning a little trip. I told her, please, to have a good one, and that it was indeed an excellent thing she was doing, seeing family and friends.

Her voice was steady and I felt under the circumstances remarkably brave. She wants nothing to do with doctors or hospitals, even though she feels her disease gnawing within her.

Her loneliness, at the edge of despair, was almost palpable even over the telephone, but so too was the fortitude that rose above it. I begged her to please call me if I could help in any way, if only to talk. She said she would, and thanked me.

I find myself filled with intense admiration for her. It is she who is being murdered by a horrible process.

And what will be her monument?

WHAT'S THAT THAT "HAPPENS"?

I do not believe, as many bumper stickers insist on telling us, that "S_ _ _ happens."

On the other hand, "Rot Is," and lives.

This is, as surely any intelligent person will allow, an altogether different matter from "S_ _ _ happens." The one looks at life from a passive I-have-been-dumped-on perspective that is not conducive to health, happiness, and well being. The other simply recognizes the hard fact that, as Hamlet put it, "merrily to the worms we go," ultimately to be sniffed out, broken down, sifted through, and recycled. Life occurs, and rot is that part of it which follows in cycles running from the almost instantaneous atomic degradation of an unstable isotope to the billions of years it takes a universe to expand and then decay. Nothing can be done about the ultimate breakdown of everything—it is the fate of us all, from isotopes to universes.

On the other hand, it seems good sport spending our particular lives in this particular galaxy trying to beat the system back in any way we can. We take comfort in the larger conceptualizations of religious faith, or for the more scientifically minded in the happy displays of nature which illustrate that from rotting ferments there invariably springs forth creation anew. The study of this process engages us now, as we glance at our universe, as much as it did Spallanzani (*animaliculae*) and Buffon (spontaneous generation) in the 18th century.

Then there is Dr. Suzuki: His reply to the "S_ _ _ happens" bumper sticker is to give every child a musical instrument. For his insight, namely, to arm kids

264

with cellos as opposed to assault weapons, he was nominated for the Nobel Prize. In music, whether worldly or "of the spheres," we find our loveliest metaphor for universal understanding and harmony. Who does not thrill to the Strauss interpretation of balance and harmony in those opening moments of the film *2001, A Space Odyssey* and how happy in contrast are those sounds to the guttural "S_ _ _ happens."

Thus do religion, science, and music refute this paltry expression once seen almost daily at any red light.

No paltry affair, on the other hand, is the noble struggle against rot. In this struggle the practice of medicine is perhaps the most distinguished of all those efforts that take a strong stand against rot. House painting, motorcycle maintenance, and the domestic arts are, of course, up there pretty well also. Having a 10-year-old and a teenager under the same roof teaches you a lot about rot perforce. My wife, whom I try to encourage from time to time when she spends so great a proportion of her energies doing laundry by saying that "this too is a meaningful beating back of rot," gives me a queer look; but even though she may wince to hear it, keeping us all reasonably hygienic deserves more credit than it gets. As for myself, lest you think I take a high and mighty position from the vantage point of being a rot–back-beating physician, I'll have you know that I am fully in charge of rot, mildew, and flea control about house and yard. Lay down your guard for a moment and rot, if it is not quite present, appears. One must take matters in hand. I, now that I am in proud possession of two shiny, new, titanium hip joints with polyethylene cups, have done so.

True, my eyes had been closed to the problems surrounding me until a recent patient rather smugly asked me to step outside my office. I did so, to watch him pull off before my very eyes a part of my siding, and with a smile tear the shingle in half with his bare hands, like cardboard, remarking that it was "rotten."

"Who put that cheap s_ _ _ on there?" he asked.

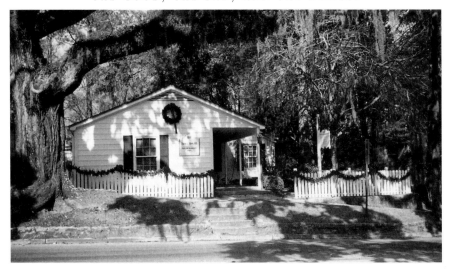

Not mildew season.

I had conveniently forgotten because, after all, that was eight years ago. He then went on to make my day by pointing out how the confederate jasmine ground cover was growing up into the walls, and coming into my waiting room. As if this were not enough, he led me around to the back of my office and pulled off a chunk of wall, showing me how the perfidious bamboo had grown up actually into the wall itself, bringing with it moisture and roaches, the former causing the wallpaper to peel away, and the latter eating the paste.

My patient left me with a sardonic chuckle. Alas! Once rot is discovered in one place, it will leap out at you from most other points of the compass.

I went inside, humbled, and immediately noticed a big stain on one of our carpets and a dying roach over in the corner, its legs feebly waving to the ceiling. And look, there was another yellowish stain down one wall, where water had run from a leaky skylight. The operating room floor looked very shabby, with a suspicious spot that might harbor a fungus or even an HIV virus. I was suddenly disgusted generally with our carpets and their industrial strength coloring.

I have taken matters in hand. I called Gorilla Builders, a local firm (not the one that did my hips) and had them come out. Of course they were horrified. They worked up an estimate. I was horrified. But what can you do?

You can go down to the bank for starters and sign a note. I have done this, and now we have basically replaced three sides of my office, installing unrottable vinyl, which I hope will be here long after I am moldy. We have pulled up all the confederate jasmine and bamboo as best we could and have a neat new landscaping. We have repainted everything, including my picket fence. We have put down beautiful carpeting of rosy red, and new wallpaper and new floors for the operating room.

The rot, for the moment, appears ostensibly gone. But I am going to keep an open and alert eye for signs of recurrence. Never again will I let all this get so out of hand. I have learned my lesson. I am wary.

It has been merely four weeks since we completed our grand refurbishment. And yet, would you believe it, as I went into the office a few days ago I saw, stimulated by our warm winter, a spike of bamboo just coming up behind the back wall, trying to find a way to grow into it again. I destroyed it in a fine frenzy.

But I confess, for an instant after that it crossed my mind that, just barely, maybe, on rare occasions, s_ _ _ does happen.

THE PHYSICIAN AS DOG

Woof! Woof!

While my new titanium hip joints and I were waiting in line at the grocery store the other day, an interesting headline in *The Sun* caught my eye. The headline came complete with a charming picture of a small pink infant, on all fours, facing the camera. His face looked exactly like our Yorkshire terrier's: a lovely muzzle, bright black button of a nose, a winning expression in the eyes, and a pink tongue delightfully ready to lick your hand in gratitude for any fragment of dog biscuit tossed his way. I was able to read just enough of the text to see that *The Sun* identified this discrepancy as the result of a "tragic incident," complete with a scandalous "hospital cover-up," and then something about "docs" rushing to volunteer their assistance.

As a matter of fact, some of the "docs" were plastic surgeons, flocking to a marvelously challenging (and charming) facial anomaly. The result was that I sheepishly bought the paper, not forgetting the other things my wife had sent me forth to fetch.

Yes, real and maybe famous plastic surgeons were even now rushing to the aid of this "dog-boy," anticipating numerous reconstructive procedures to rid him of his fur and restore a "soft and supple human skin," all surrounded by a tremendous outpouring of emotion on the part of the population at large.

The hospital, on the other hand, clearly had attempted a massive cover-up of this incident. But *The Sun's* keen investigative reporters had blown the lid on this subterfuge, and found that somehow or other dog sperm had gotten mixed up with human sperm in the central sperm bank.

What a tragedy indeed! You would think that some central government agency, or at least local bureaucracy, would have in place provisions for not allowing such kinds of carelessness! And what, I thought to myself, for goodness sake is this hospital doing with dog sperm anyway? Is there some deeper plot afoot? Is the American Hospital Association trying to pull some sort of fast one on us? Are we going to the dogs?

It was not a long step from these questions to a recollection of the superb editorial by the editor of the *Journal of The Florida Medical Association*, Dr. Jacques Caldwell, that I had recently read. It was he who drew our attention to the machinations of the American Hospital Association's platform, which in summary is one of gaining as absolutely as possible hegemony not only over the delivery of medicine, but as well over the physicians who do the delivering. As I reread Dr. Caldwell's editorial, it became clear to me that hospitals and the powers that run them would quite clearly, and without scruple, be happy to see us as dogs to their masters. They would be glad to transmute us, I do hazard to guess, into furry creatures kept beneath their groaning table, and to whom they might throw a crust or bit of bone for which we would yap gratefully, thankful for whatever we got.

But surely I dramatize. Maybe it is simply the mere artiste in my system, exaggerating for media effect. Forgive me; I must bring myself down to earth and reality. And so I shall.

Up here in little old Tallahassee, as the rain falls ceaselessly, we are presently once again about to engage with our hospital. On the other hand maybe not; maybe the hospital will simply be delighted to accept all of the provisions we have inserted into our new Bylaws.

Do you know about Bylaws? These are a lot of words that in essence have a certain binding quality, and I think even contractual validity under the law as stated by Florida courts. Our Bylaws, perhaps like others, have been sadly neglected, become out of date and in fact mere anachronisms in the face of postmodern attitudes towards medical care. Our Bylaws used to simply state that physicians did such and such, and should behave in this or that manner, and that everything would be fine. Recently, since the attempt by the hospital to discharge one of our respected radiotherapists, solely on the basis of "economic credentialing" as far as anyone can see, this and other not dissimilar stimuli have provoked us toward looking more closely into protecting our rights within the hospital. For example, what is the point of being allowed hospital "privileges" if you are denied use of the hospital equipment? Such points, and numerous others, never entered into our previous consideration, nor would have been dreamt of by sane people 10 years ago. Now they have become crucial.

Our new Bylaws are written with the hope that we shall maintain some degree of autonomy and security in our hospital practices. We are very pointedly demanding that on no account shall a qualified physician, of good professional and ethical standing, have his or her hospital privileges brought to closure by others who possess merely business degrees and associated ulterior motives. We have had much advice from respected legal firms, even from way up north. We have what we think is a good document.

As documents go, it expresses one opinion, namely, that of the medical staff, and will doubtless be weighed in the balance against the counter opinions of the hospital administration. Most of the time it makes good sense that areas should be found capable of negotiation and compromise. I am sure there will be points within our new Bylaws where such areas exist. On the other hand it will be important to be steadfast, recognizing there are also areas that must be nonnegotiable if we are to survive, at least other than as dogs struggling amongst ourselves for whatever poor bones the hospital may toss us, or fawning upon the hospital in the hope that we may be sufficiently favored to be tossed a kibble or two.

Dog physicians we must not be!

And if the hospitals think they can infiltrate us in some strange way by using dog sperm, I say "well done!" to *The Sun* for exposing these cruel and perfidious tactics. Let us stand up for our freedom and humanity!

And down with dog sperm in our hospitals!

WHILE WE'RE AT IT...

I am regarding it as a singular experiment that we should have had two attorneys, male and female at that, running our country. Now, finally, we have been allowed the insightful experience of two lawyers messing around in our lives from the very tippy top of the pinnacles of national power, shining down upon ourselves who are struggling to make a living. Not since Nixon and Ford (the one resigning, the other never elected) have we had a lawyer as president, and now that we have had two it has been not only singular but almost thrilling. The question, however, yet remains: Can, should, lawyers run a government?

Of course in this instance we can take comfort in the fact that we have not been led into the future by two mere attorneys, but rather two Yale attorneys. With the possible exception of those presidents who graduated from Harvard Law School, what could be better? One of them, even, was first and the other fourth in their graduating class! And it seems to me I have heard that Bill (I'm not sure about Hillary) has read *Moby Dick* without even skipping those long, dreary passages about flensing blubber from the poor whale. But, I would rather not think about that, because there is yet a little time for it to cross Bill's mind that what is good for whales might be good for us, just as a finishing touch in his final year.

Let me add that when it comes to Yale, if not *Moby Dick*, I know of what I speak. In medical school one of my best friends was a Yalie. He was something of a delightful person: tall, handsome, urbane but down to earth. He also had, as part of his Yale background, a slight but interesting curl to his nostril which gave him the look and something of the style of a Regency Beau. He would have been a good model for a paperback cover to one of Georgette Heyer's novels, a "hero" who might with debonair sangfroid, the sun coming up in the east, coolly look down the barrel of a dueling pistol and drill you dead with compassion, afterwards repairing to a local inn to have kippers and a glass of port. Duels being forbidden by the early 1960s, he drove a Porsche instead, and dated a young lady as suitable as himself for inclusion in the Georgette Heyer scenario. They married, indeed, and lived happily ever after because he became a dermatologist.

But I was speaking of the slight curl to his nostril. It was subtle and marvelously enhancing. I don't think he had it before he went to Yale. He could elevate his ala (*levator superioris alaeque nasi)* ever so slightly with the barest trace of a "sniff." On him it was attractive and nothing supercilious.

In certain of her pictures, on the other hand, I note that Mrs. Clinton also has a faint flair of nostril, but unlike David's case hers has no humor. Surely she too learned nostril expanding techniques at Yale because it is part of what they teach there, I think particularly in the second year of law school, but she does not control it quite so well as my friend, or for that matter William Buckley, who learned it in their more plastic undergraduate years. I have the terrible feeling that behind closed doors in the White House Mrs. Clinton practices alar flaring in possibly libertine fashion, and particularly on Bill, who, being from sturdy Arkansas stock, does not have the power over his nostril, and other bits of anatomy too, which his wife possesses. His nasal skin, as any acute diagnostician will notice, is slightly thickened with just a touch of sebaceous hypertrophy necessarily resulting in a less mobile member. It may put him at a certain disadvantage when Hillary and he discuss policy. I have, of course, in all likelihood wandered; but those of you who understand the importance of subtle signs will forgive me.

The straightforward facts are that we have almost survived a delicate period wherein two lawyers, the best trained our country can produce, have done their best to decide for us physicians our fate. In fairness may I not propose a view of how our government should treat attorneys?

More specifically I propose the following: First, that all lawyers be simply paid by the government $40 to $50 an hour, plus expenses, but carefully monitored to see that they are actually at their desks on task. An appropriate bureaucracy should be set up to approve, tabulate, issue, and double check remuneration, to be called henceforth the Legal Care Finance Administration (LCFA), next door to HCFA,[1] so that these two bureaucracies can bowl against each other on Friday nights. We should immediately write documents amounting to thousands of pages, minutely describing to the lawyers what they can and cannot do. Honesty and integrity should be carefully defined and coded in a particularly bureaucratic way, citing all current and historical references, these definitions to be enforced by appropriate penalties with interest naturally included where convenient.

We should also write a manifesto that it should be an inherent right for all Americans to have legal care readily available rather than as an all too expensive privilege. This right should include all classes of society, including even physicians. The enormous cost of legal "care" as it is presently constituted, a cost so high and so hidden that no one has dared calculate its true dimension, must be brought severely under control by ways and means that any decent bureaucrat can discover. Physicians, who may know no more about the law than lawyers know about the practice of medicine, should clearly devise these ways and means. We should not allow demur from the American Bar Association which, after all, is nothing more than representative of a gigantic vested interest.

Yes, of course, some feathers may be ruffled, but like gentlemen and gentlewomen let us hope we can settle these issues without exciting professional antipathies. Still, human nature being what it is, the lawyers are likely to get

---

[1]Health Care Finance Administration, about which I can write no further.

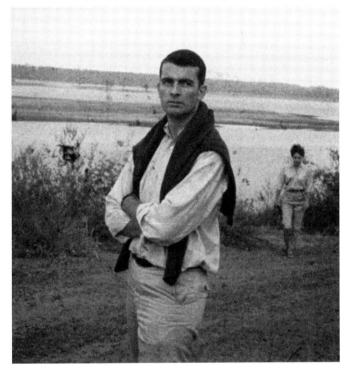

David Payne as I knew him then.

angry, particularly because they are so highly trained in contention and confrontation. If they insist on becoming really irritated or even mean, I then propose a straightforward one-on-one duel, each side pledging afterwards to put aside past rancor. Yes, at dawn some morning on a green field, when the mist is rising over the river, let their lawyer appear and our physician.

As our man I nominate Dr. David Payne, Yale, '60. Let them duel, nostrils aquiver.

Afterwards, for no one will hit the mark, let us all go have eggs McMuffin and O.J. at McDonalds, and our two professions live happily ever after, our petty differences settled in the happy recognition that the sick will be treated, Justice and Truth served, and a pretty penny saved for the country we love.

FINALLY, A SORT OF SOLUTION

I realize that all of you have been eagerly awaiting my solution to the "Health-care-cost-containment-delivery" crisis. Yes, I know that I was supposed to come out with my program before now, but did not, to the great disappointment of many. You must, after all, allow that this is a knotty problem of Gordian proportions, a lot worse than what happens when your suture material gets looped around itself and your needle holder, and then gets caught up in your fingers, and maybe around your neck or the ear of your surgical assistant. No, that is nothing compared to the knottiness of the health-care issues I have been so seriously thinking about.

Well, finally, here it is, like it or not, my very own solution.

It has been curious to me, as something of an aside, that our government, "for the people, by the people" and "at the people" (as Oscar Wilde defined "democracy") has not called me before one of our government committees to give testimony regarding my attitudes toward health care and its costs. On the other hand I don't feel particularly offended because better folk than I have been snubbed with worse singularity.

After all, I fully understand that simply nothing should be allowed to interfere with bureaucratic process, and the fact that physicians may know something special about health care might clearly serve to confuse the bureaucratic issues and greater concerns. I hate being cynical, and do so only for fun, but I have a suspicion that were God himself to appear before a senate subcommittee in His or Her role as "The Great Physician" even His (Her) words would be suspect as coming from the mind of someone with a "vested interest," inevitable bias, and egregiously self-serving, naturally. No, Divinity itself would go unheard, because Divinity clearly does not know much about the numerous panaceas inherent in due bureaucratic process. If Divinity did the world would not, after all, be so terribly full of flaws, would it?

Lacking any hope, however, of appearing before a committee, permit me therefore to take advantage of this homely platform to state my remedies for health care, and most particularly its cost containment. It is an antibureau-cratic remedy and, therefore, frowned upon by those august powers, but I think you will agree with me that it would work quite nicely.

My solution, crudely put, is simply to mandate that the practice of med-icine be performed after the fashions and practices of a date in time no later than December 31, 1954.

Instead of that noxious green, giving undue dignity to the color of "bile," surgeons would wear white again. Nurses would be (good fun!) rather more deferential, and even in awe of physicians on their rounds; they would maybe even wear red crosses on their aprons and little hats. There would be no ICUs, but we would have antibiotics and even steroids. Waiting rooms would be full of hard seats made of plastic and chrome, and the waiting period would be long and dreary, but one must give up something after all. Syringes would be made of glass and needles sterilized and used over and over again (cost-effective that), accepting the inconvenience of an occasional barb on the point, but with the much enhanced safety factor resulting from the fact that there would be no silicone coatings on them which, of course, we need to get rid of anyway. True, we would not have beepers vibrating in our hip pockets, but perhaps there would be some compensation in having the movie you might be attending sud-denly interrupted, and an announcement flashed on the screen: "Would Dr. Blank please call such and such a number." People would see the shadowy fig-ure of "us" as we wearily arose from our seat to answer the call of the needy, and know that, yes, there goes good old Dr. Blank once more on an errand of mercy, and whisper to each other about the nobility of medicine's purpose.

Marvelous for us, as well, would be the fact that for all practical purposes there would be no known governmental structure overseeing the medical community, this in itself saving a vast amount of dollars. And yet, thanks to the perception of the government and public seeing us leave the movie theater so gracefully, the government and population at large would look up to and trust fully the integrity of the medical establishment.

There would, of course, be essentially no medico-legal issues, saving, perhaps more than for any other reason, an enormous amount of time, effort, and money. The young people who now go to law school would instead pursue military careers, or become foresters or farmers, with even the odd artist among them, but all to the nation's better advantage. Medicine, or more accurately, its technology, would not be so complex or costly as to demand any need for its "rationing," and death would generally be expected as an ultimate outcome of, after all, life.

Of course, we would not be able to put every little bitty wound that looks problematic into HBO[1] chambers on a twice-daily basis for weeks on end, but maybe after a few days or weeks most might heal anyway. And no, we would not be getting CT scans on everyone with a headache out of fear of litigation otherwise. Nor would we have the laser and all it stands for in the name of a space age "ray," but life would still go on.

Everyone in 1954, after all, was living and dying, and on the whole (I remember it!) accepting of that state of affairs as being pretty irresistible.

---

[1]Hyperbaric oxygen, which is to say the chamber in which oxygen is compressed, and wherein concurrently is placed the patient who one hopes does not suffer from claustrophobia. Such chambers are enormously useful, life-saving indeed, for divers suffering from the "bends," but because most of us do not get the "bends," and I think even fewer in 1954, its utilization until recently was thought to be a good deal less than "occasional." Like all technology, and more rapidly if it catches the eye of the Media, its use for more than what it is good for merely awaits "discovery." Suddenly every hospital must have one, and to pay for it honest folk find that it is good not only for the "bends" but also "hangnails" and everything in between. At considerable cost.

Perhaps we are more demanding now, but could not the government, at small expense and by merely suggesting that you would be audited by the IRS if you did otherwise, mount an effective campaign that would teach us once more to put up with a few inconveniences?

Well, the people on dialysis might not like it, nor the people looking to have their coronary arteries cleaned out, nor the ones dying who might otherwise be cured of Hodgkin's disease. And, oh dear, suddenly I think of a wonderful friend who recently had open heart surgery, and is almost magically restored to us and his family. And the very nice gentleman I met the other day in my office who had a kidney transplant many years ago and has flourished. And worse, though I struggle to suppress the thought, what about my lovely titanium hip joints of which I am so proud?

Drat!

So much for back to the future! No wonder I am never asked to testify to anything.

AT LEAST THEY DON'T DRINK

The biggest trouble with the computer is that it lacks sensitivity. What it does well it simply flaunts, leaving those of us who are not mathematical idiot-savants belittled in comparison. It is all the more infuriating in that it gives us not even a passing glance of credit for those things we may do quite well, and which it cannot even begin to comprehend, like watching a sunset or eating an ice cream cone.

The computer in our office, which I have borne up with patiently for two years, is as smug as they come. It is a Xenix[1] system, which means it is altogether too big for its own britches. Superior though it thinks itself, it is nonetheless perfectly capable of nasty screw-ups for which it offers no apology whatsoever. Real human beings, however, people who should be using their time and energies towards more poetic goals, are nonetheless required to spend sometimes hours on the telephone trying to get in touch with some other computer, somewhere, that will tell us what is wrong and how to placate our own instrument.

It is set in its ways, and positively refuses to behave in a sensitive manner even towards my friends. I am thinking of one who is a classical musician, but a little bit poor and therefore without health insurance. I relieved him of a mole, or something like, and even though we have repeatedly told the computer not to bill him every month, my friend, who is very sensitive, calls in alarm at the receipt of yet another bill. No matter how many times

---

[1] I have no idea what this is, and am not even sure I can spell it.

I have told him to tear the bill into tiny shreds, he now has misgivings about me, thinking I am only saying that, and the reality is that pretty soon the computer is going to knock on his door and break his piano-playing fingers if he does not pay up. The computer simply doesn't *care*.

For a while I thought it was all my fault, and that maybe I would have to make an appointment for our computer and me to have a joint session with some shrink or psychologist versed in "relationship therapy." But now that the great HRS computer scandal has come to light, particularly filling the pages of our local newspaper, I see that I am not alone in feeling discouraged about maintaining a mutually reciprocating and caring relationship with our Xenix. As everyone knows, the HRS Super computer sent out checks totaling millions of dollars to people whose names and addresses it more or less made up, or forgot to forget, (even when told, maybe) with someone on the receiving end of the line nonetheless ready to take advantage of the opportunity and cash in. In the final analysis, I'm not sure anyone is quite capable, ultimately, of knowing what any computer may be up to.

Which brings me to another, but related, point. The computer may be simply wonderful at lots of things, and without it we would never have a definition of pi to a few million places. But I think it is directly to blame for the upsurge in the inability to get an intelligent answer from a human being when you call some agency or acronym with a mild question. You know what I mean. You have a question about your tax return or a Medicare account. You call the ever-available 800 number and get someone who knows absolutely nothing, but who transfers you to someone else who knows nothing, who transfers you to someone who knows nothing even more, and refers you back to the original number you called. People know "nothing" now because in their offices they think the computer has done everything and, therefore, no more need be said or thought, and they go home content with a good day's work.

I have a patient, for example, who the other day regaled me at length regarding her embarrassment and even pain that she had repetitively

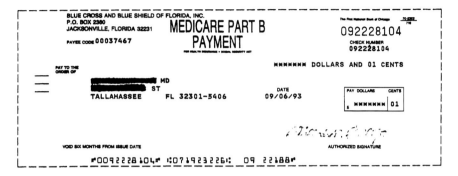

received from a laboratory a notice of a balance due, which amounted to a considerable sum. She had given to everyone she thought necessary the information that she had a secondary policy to cover costs above and beyond Medicare's allowance for such services, but the computer could not have cared less almost by definition. Finally the computer wrote her a truly nasty letter, saying that she would be attacked by fierce lawyers and all the dignities of the courts unless she coughed up. A most mild lady of the older school, she was finally forced to have a little fit, and after a tedious experience got through to someone responsible who happily took care of it, blandly noting that she should not have worried, "because it was only the computer." The moral of this story is that if someone, like in olden times, had been dealing with her account, following it along, getting accustomed to it, writing it down in a great ledger with a feather pen, that person would have in all likelihood known what was going on. The computer separates one from any intimacy whatsoever with an account.

In other words, the computer lacks any chance of discernment. I have actually seen, with my own eyes, a check sent to one of our local doctors from Medicare which deserves publishing, particularly at this delicate moment when the government is affirming the prospect of new efficiency in the bureaucracy of health care. The check was in payment to the doctor for services rendered. After everything disallowed was subtracted, his services were worth exactly one cent. Such a check lacks discernment and could even be construed as a touch insulting; on the other hand I am willing to allow that this particular computer, clearly not a Xenix, might have had an anomalous sense of humor.

Of course, even people who use pens, with real ink, can make an occasional interesting "mistake." I think of a young man I know, who some years ago was in his teens and desperately trying to save enough money to go to Europe. Among other commendable activities, he drove a taxi for one summer. A well-known local lawyer, indeed a veritable judge who lived in a town east of us, called requesting taxi services. The judge, who liked to do his drinking in Tallahassee for some reason, on this inebriated occasion still had the sense to know he had better not try driving home. So Mark took him, and without glancing at it put the check that the judge wrote him in his pocket. When he got home and looked at it, he saw that it was made out for $1,500,000 and no cents. Neatly signed. Mark never called him on it, so the judge got home free.

It was just the kind of thing a lawyer . . . or a computer too . . . would do, isn't it?

CHOOSING MY COLORS

I would never ordinarily look at the yellow pages of a telephone book. Mostly, I don't want to see all the pictures of chiropractors, nor read their claims, nor their impassioned notices to the public that they are this and that and, of course, accept payment plans—anything whatsoever that will cough up a buck. I don't want to see their bland expressions gazing forth at me as though to condemn a terrible back injury, and a slipped cervical disc to boot, about which I know lamentably nothing. Nor do I want to see how they have preempted us by the fact that their job description begins with a "C" and ours a "P"; and so they achieve a subtle lead over us by their placement in the yellow pages.

I confess also that I do not particularly want to see my small name lost in the fine print between the larger notifications of other MDs. I don't want to have to compare how telephonically diminutive is my standing with my colleagues. Perhaps I am too noncompetitive or simply have not attended enough "medical merchandising" seminars. Allowing that point, I equally allow myself the feeling, maybe out of joint, that something kind of garish is happening even to us in little ol' Tallahassee in the telephone listings.

It is not, by the way, my fault that I write this. I would have gone on quite happily, like a cross between an ostrich and a clam, had not our new and improved yellow pages been pointed out to me, and by no less a luminary than Dr. Terry McCoy himself, now the veritable President-Elect of the Florida Medical Association and handshaker of not only Bob Dole, but also former President Bush (and who knows whom else?).

The point was noted by Dr. McCoy as I was enjoying one of my now and again proctoscopic examinations, when he, pleasant chit-chatterer that he is, brought up these insidious, possibly invidious yellow pages. He said that he has become an aficionado not only of our very own yellow pages but those elsewhere, finding them a kind of entertaining read, and discovering in them suggestive hints regarding the present state of medicine and portents for its future.

The exam completed, and I restored to a modicum of decency, Dr. McCoy insisted on fetching the latest telephone directory, hot off the press, forcing me to look, or otherwise prescribing for me a full colonoscopy with the light aperitif of a gallon of GoLYTELY beforehand. I was titillated to discover that we Tallahassee physicians are now presenting ourselves in living technicolor, and/or other eye-catching announcements, not quite yet extravaganzas. Of course, despite these timid "advances," we still have a lot to learn from the chiropractors, who probably chuckle in what I suppose is their beer over our naivety and backwardness. Certainly, for the most part, so we may still appear, but some of us are coming quite along, I thought.

Such lovely reds, such handsome blues, and here and there pictures and scattered renderings of how marvelous are our qualifications, how much we do and can do; how much, it seems to me by implication, better we probably are than our erstwhile peers and colleagues. Forgive me the use of the term "erstwhile." But in the "new" yellow pages, now blazing with neon color, it seems to me we diminish our professional relationship with our peers, who become herein frank "competitors." Beyond this sorry fact, of course, is the further one that when you speak of "competition" and "markets" what you are really speaking of is "money." Yet we claim, at least to the government and the public, that it is "patient care" that matters. The yellow pages seem to belie this image of idealism and service. But then, of course, there are always excuses and rationalizations, subtle issues that this article does not address; and after all the writer of it may be on the veritable brink of fuddy-duddyism.

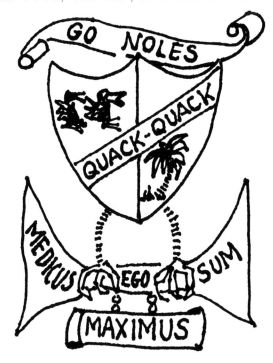

Fantasy for a full page color telephone ad.

Nonetheless there is something a bit sad about it all. Do the yellow pages announce the cutting edge of our future? Will we be forced to advertise our "wares" like the quacks of yore? Who knows? Maybe this year the telephone company simply had a wonderful "merchandiser" of its own. Maybe next year the yellow pages will be yellow again, and our names simply stated in black, doing what we do.

Of course, "doing what we do," even in color, may not be sufficient for the brave new world of modern medicine. Here in Tallahassee the great marketing strategem would be to align myself, if only by the least tangential implication, to the FSU football team.

I stretch my memory to recall if I have ever treated a real FSU football player, so I could then call myself "Plastic Surgeon to the Seminoles." But no one comes to mind . . . but wait! I did once treat the wife of a player! Won't that do? Or I could build a new office in the shape of a football. It is this sort of thing that enhances prestige and of course cash-flow analysis, but because I am philosophically incapable of such a leap, even if I could discover an architect who was, I must settle for less.

Perhaps, more modestly, and without redesigning my office to look like a football, I could list myself in the yellow pages as simply "The Seminole Plastic Surgery Institute." But then do I set myself up for Letters to the Editor raging against me for the ill-appropriation of the name of a proud Native American nation? Our own government and judicial system are enough of a threat without having the Creeks rise against me too!

No, bright nonpartisan colors are for me quite enough to cogitate for the present. Maybe I will bloom into a whole page of them next year because no one seems much offended.

But I simply will not stand for . . . and draw the line in my committal against . . . fuchsia!

Just color me, mostly, puce.

DECORUM IN
REBUS ADVERSIS

I know only a minuscule amount of Latin but enjoy imagining that somehow or other I am facile in this ancient language. It gives a kind of gravitas to any remarks one might otherwise all too casually make, and has a resonance far better than simply piping up, in a wee shrill voice, "decorum in adversity!"

The "adversity," of course, relates to the onslaughts the practice of medicine is facing and has yet to face. Like most of us good, bad, and homely folk, I need every prop possible to maintain some semblance of decorum when the chips are down. My mother used to tell me I was one of those perfectly horrid children who wanted everything in the toy store, and when I didn't get it, I would fall down on the floor and beat my limbs and head against it, howling. I don't think I was ever spanked, although in those days before the micromanagement of our social ways and means it was quite permissible, and might have forced upon me a better ability to be graceful under pressure.

As it is, I find it easy to be marvelously gracious when I am the recipient of little accolades, small honors, and toys. In return, I can benignly reradiate a graceful *noblesse oblige*, put on the face of modesty, and return the compliment. It's when the chips are down that the maintenance of poise becomes a more intriguing challenge, as anyone quite knows.

My perspective, of course, is highly parochial, but as I observe our local social scene from within the narrow confines of the surgeon's lounge just off the operating suite, where all bon vivants gather from 11:30 to 2:00 to eat the hospital fare brought us on a trolley, well-laced with

Tabasco sauce, on the whole, I think we are bearing up right well as a profession. True, there is beneath the surface an undercurrent of despair, and a good deal of gallows humor is bandied about here and there as we look towards our future, or conceivably the lack of it. Rumor and innuendo run rampant, and there is a certain amount of eye-rolling, if not quite yet hand-wringing, as we contemplate things like government health plans and HMOs.

Beyond these old "saws," however, we are slightly taken aback when someone notes that the nurses are reported to be presenting a bill to the Florida Legislature that will allow them not only to diagnose but to prescribe for various and sundry diseases. We are interested, as well, to observe how our local IPA, or HMO, or other acronym, struggles to stay afloat as it is caught up in these mighty waters rushing us somewhere. We note how the optometrists, at least in Virginia, are now licensed to perform surgery, maybe even C-sections! And yet, ostensibly, we MDs remain a fairly merry bunch, perhaps regarding the circumstances surrounding us rather as those people who live on that tiny shore between the sea and Mount Stromboli regard new smoke rising from their volcano's crater.

At least we have not yet, to my knowledge, descended into overt, internecine viciousness, despite my remarks about the "yellow pages." Our "cool," or our "decorum," yet remains intact in Tallahassee. This is more than can be said for some areas of the country.

Let me note, for example, the recent incident in Worcester, Massachusetts, its decorum (after all, it is almost Boston) shattered by a headline that said "Doctors Fined for Fight in Operating Room." Apparently neurosurgeon Dr. K. and anesthesiologist Dr. K.C., succumbing to these harsh times, did as I used to do in the dime store. The news clipping related that Dr. K.C. actually swore at Dr. K. who then—get this—"threw a cotton-tipped applicator at Dr. K.C." It is not divulged whether the Q-tip hit Dr. K.C. with its cotton end or wooden, but Dr. K.C. had quite enough of this and "the two then raised their fists and scuffled briefly, at one point wrestling on the floor. A nurse monitored the anesthetized patient as the doctors fought."

Well, this is all mighty disturbing to one's sense of decorum, and Miss Manners, if she has anything to say about etiquette in the OR, would probably deplore these actions in no uncertain terms. At least, although this can be no justification, the article notes that "afterwards, the doctors resumed the half-hour-long operation." Good for them, at that, and what is wrong with letting out a few frustrations at an early point in time before worse tensions accumulate? True, one does not throw a Q-tip at someone lightly, but it is better than a #11 scalpel blade or an anesthesia machine. Indeed, if we would all throw Q-tips at each other rather than spraying ourselves with 9-mm missiles, etc., we would be the better for it.

In any case these kinds of episodes illustrate the temper of our times. Nerves are frayed. Emotions lie nearer the surface. We are all, after all, about to become employees of either the government or a "friendly" HMO, God help us, a fate we all went into medicine at least in part to escape.

And yet hope springs eternal, doesn't it? And who knows what good can come of it? Perhaps we are going to become more thoughtful, like true volcano-lovers, and less smug. We may regard ourselves more as a part of the real universe. For example, one of our most highly respected surgeons, whom you would not particularly expect to be an avid Stephen Hawking enthusiast, brought up unprompted the subject of Hawking in the surgeons' lounge! I was astonished, and yet saw in his remarks a deeper search for life's meaning, for metaphysical value, for verities that are the true basics upon which the ability of each of us to survive in society must be based. Who knows where such undertakings might lead?

But meanwhile, we cannot help but expect and anticipate that there will be further outbreaks, not only among surgeons, but even among internists too, and conceivably perhaps even psychiatrists will suffer lapses.

Let us, therefore, be on guard against these trends. We are going to have to be all the more graceful and gracious to ourselves, to our colleagues, and to our patients. Let us, indeed, bear ourselves in such fashion that if, were our profession yet to last a thousand years, men and women then, as yet unborn (of course!) shall say . . .

THIS WAS THEIR FINEST HOUR!

THE COMPLEXITY
OF IGNORANCE

I f we were perfectly simple, perfectly all encompassing, and perfectly all knowing, we might be almost God, or at least that
white light that came out of the spaceship at the end of *E.T.*

But we ain't any of that. As the poet neatly put it, "Life, like a dome
of many colored glass, stains the white radiance of eternity." Worse! For
"many colored" we might even substitute "murky."

Lacking clarity, therefore, we take to drink, and condone bureaucrats in
their passage of hundreds of thousands of laws telling us how to behave. Our
ignorance, maybe, can be quietly camouflaged behind the veil of law,
whether it regulates how doctors are to behave or gravity is to operate.

You will perceive that I write this as we more or less complete the leg-
islative session here in Tallahassee. I am trying from within the ivory-towered
security of our living room (a cat in my lap and a martini in hand) to be forgiving of our elected officials, politicos, bureaucrats, rabble-rousers, lobby-
ists, media moguls, and minions of the "Politically Correct." After all, if I am
not at least a wee bit forgiving of their obfuscation, as they muddy the
waters of the simple practice of healing, how can I forgive myself?

And so, I sit here, martini in hand, cat in lap, pontificating to my wife
with the best of the politicians and, for that matter as well, quite as
obscurely. I have just made the most elaborate analogy, betwixt olives fished
forth from my martini, between the various and almost innumerable regulatory agencies that interject their ways and means upon the practice of
medicine and the tediously detailed, burdensomely officious, and highly

refined processes of medieval scholasticism. In those days, if you varied a certain iota from received opinion, it would land you at the stake or on the rack in the hands of an inquisition.

If you think I said this as simply as that, you are wrong. By the time I got it all out, the cat had jumped from my lap, and the hideous thought had crossed my consciousness that maybe, despite all, I should have been a politician! What a dizzying and dizzy linguistic display! What *non sequiturs*! No cat, of course, would put up with such nonsense.

My wife does not get so carried away. If there is anyone, thank God, who is a "white light" in our family it is she. "What in the world did all that mean?" she asked me, lovingly and with the sweet tolerance born of a generous spirit.

"Oh dear," thought I, "I am going to have to do this all over again." Happily, my wife was saved from a second dose of philosophizing by our daughter Meredith coming in, she of the muddy sneakers without laces, to inquire about dinner. Relieved, I gave in saying, "Oh, it's all just too complex, isn't it?" knocking off my last olive. But my eyes, like Clint Eastwood before he does something nasty, narrowed; and I thought that I just might spare my wife and instead subject this essay to these ruminations instead. Ha!

So here I am demonstrating in the simplest, most concise manner conceivable how ignorance breeds complexity. Perhaps this point is self-evident, and we all perfectly well know it, and there is nothing much we can do about it; but that doesn't mean we can't kind of marvel at it, as I am doing here. We remain in a bewildering universe that provides us only glimpses of answers, and sometimes those prove wrong because there are plenty of "trick" questions. In our ignorance, we develop concepts into which we force the facts to fit, raising up rulers and electing officials who will pass laws to make sure we toe the line. Once the concept is in place, and all the trouble taken to fabricate the rules and regulations ordaining its *modus operandi*, we cling to it for dear life.

I know wonderfully little about medieval scholasticism, except that it was ingenious in arguing the finer points of a beautifully conceptualized cosmology. Although we use different words and have our own syntax, the debate is still often enough of how many angels can stand on the head of a pin. But how grand now seem the medieval arguments, performed in the impeccable Latin of Aquinas; how grand the poetry of their concerns even if expressed in the vulgar tongue, but that tongue the *terza rima* of Dante. We, in struggling with our own ignorance, denied the purging fire of the 7th Cornice of Purgatory, embed ourselves less elegantly but with equal intensity in systems of thought at least of equivalently incomprehensible subtlety. We cling to them, of course, for dear life; it is, after all, all we have; why embrace the upstart Copernicus, anyway, when with a little fiddling Ptolemy can yet be forced to work?

More germane to our moment are quarks, the angels of our system. As the great physicist Murray Gell-Mann said while expostulating on the recent discovery of "The Top Quark," our own version of the biggest angel on the pin head, "Not finding it would have been shocking . . . it would have been an inconceivable disaster for theorists if they could not find it." Now that we have trapped this veritable Quark of quarks I can guarantee you we are damn well going to do everything possible to keep it. To lose it would be as disastrous as saying, in the 15th century, that the earth goes around the sun.

Keeping systems intact at least creates a business opportunity for the professional enforcers. In medicine alone we have them aplenty, never mind in a more general sense the (then) inquisition and the IRS (now) to whom we give such powers of regulation and oversight. The guidelines, as they are going to come down to us in the up and coming *Great Book of Rules and Regulations for the Practice of Medicine and the Delivery of Healthcare in the Good Old U.S. of A.* may be slightly different from those of medieval conception. I do not think we will be liable to being burned alive in front of a merry crowd; yet I also think there will be refined means, and it might as well be written in Latin or Greek, of seeing to it that doctors learn what small fry we are within the cosmological scheme now in process of invention by politicians and bureaucrats.

Thus, as I see it, out of ignorance must be devised elaborate systems, the more the merrier. They do good services camouflaging our lack of knowledge.

If my wife were to read this, for I do not regale her with suggesting she do so, I wonder if she would find my trumpetings more comprehensible this time around? As I said at the beginning, it is this sort of exposition that drives one to martinis and too many olives. Better, let me add, the nice soft purring of a neutered, fluffy, white cat in your lap, from whom one can maybe learn a little grace.

In any case, I sigh, let me indeed count my blessings. As St. Francis nicely put it, cutting through all the bureaucracy and red tape and letting the angels fall where they may,

Laudate et benedicete, mi Signore et rengratiate et servitele
con grande humilitate.

Which is to say, of course, give thanks and be (just a little) humble; and if you are more into quarks than prayer, as new systems of health care are thrust upon us, you might at least keep your fingers crossed.

It worked for Copernicus, who probably said some prayers himself. They didn't, after all, burn him alive.

[AN EDITORIAL COMMENT]

I have never been very sure just what Editors do.

In my 10 years or so of being editor (that is a very small "e" by the way) of our local medical society newsletter, I have experienced very little to illuminate the yet arcane nature of a real Editor's role.

I scarcely know what to think when I think of an Editor: perhaps of Maxwell Perkins, who deserves a lot of credit for discovering a variety of big literary pickles like Marjorie Kinnan Rawlings, F. Scott Fitzgerald, and most particularly Thomas Wolfe. Respecting this latter, Perkins as Editor was rather more of an archeologist, unearthing trunkfuls of Wolfe's writings in confused and well-nigh hopeless disarray, and putting them together for the world to admire. Without Perkins, Wolfe might not have made it, but this is editing at its most rarefied and is scarcely worth our consideration here.

On a more mundane level, I think I think that Editors by some miraculous means know a lot about grammar and Henry Watson Fowler, both the British and American usage; I think for some reason they know where commas ought and ought not to go; and like Hamlet (I believe it was) can more or less tell a hawk from a handsaw and the difference between running a gamut and doing a gambit. Somehow or other, a good Editor is subtle and maybe even a bit shrewd; somehow or other, at their best, they are creatures who are willing to give thoughtfulness a real try, not only for themselves but more remarkably allowing it in others, even going so far as to encourage it. Theirs is, often enough, a thankless task in which they gracefully hand out accolades while receiving few enough.

A good Editor must be able to walk a fine line, neatly balanced, and always aware that those most simple life-giving substances, for example, earth, air, fire, and water, are in truth almost beyond comprehension, complex and rendered all the more so when mixed up in various ways.

Editors must avoid being silly, even the editor of *MAD* magazine. On the other hand, just as an example, editors can clearly slip up. Perhaps it is only from my perspective as a physician that the other day I considered the remarks of Ms. Ellen Levine, then the editor of *Redbook* magazine, only slightly better than frankly fatuous. Perhaps they were merely flatuous, for which I would simply have to forgive her because I do it all the time.

In any case, I was idling away an idle moment when *Redbook* fell into my lap. I opened it and saw Ms. Levine's picture hard by her column, "The Editor's Notes." The picture caught my eye, being that of, I suppose, a handsome lady who has contrived the most attractive look of a whimsical villain but, with her hair alternately streaked white and black looking, not to get overly personal (a temptation always spurned by good, real Editors), remarkably like an interesting zebra.

For those of you who do not recall the May 1994 issue of *Redbook*, I can only say you might enjoy it. There are certainly nice articles, which I passed over, describing "What Loni did for Love . . . at Last the Truth behind the Betrayal" and on "What Other Women Will (and Won't) Do in Bed" and about how stress is possibly damaging your skin. There is nothing in this issue on silicone, which possibly cost the magazine a good deal in terms of sales that month, but you can't have everything all the time. We had, however, Ms. Levine's comments about AIDS. Actually she started her editorial addressing the pleasures of Mother's Day, which led me on because I am delighted with that occasion despite my being a father. Mother's Day was merely a gambit, if not a gamut, used merely as a gimmick to harangue us with the following comment, to wit, "as you think about what you would like to receive this Mother's Day, remember also what you want to send: a card to Congress calling for an end to the AIDS crisis."

Maybe, I thought, while Congress was conjuring up the ever newer and more improved version of that corpus which will soon descend upon us, hereinafter called *The Grandiose Set of Rules, Regulations, and Enactments, Designed to Bring Safe, Sane, and Perfecto Medical Care to Every United States Citizen and Why Not Our Dogs?*, why not tag onto this bill a simple rider ending the AIDS crisis? This seems to be what Ms. Levine thinks Congress should do.

Perhaps I simply don't agree with Ms. Levine that in legislation lies some panacea. I do not think you can browbeat research into coming up with a solution to the HIV virus, which is a great deal more clever than anyone in Congress anyway. As a real Editor, indeed an editor at a very pinnacle of power, I suppose Ms. Levine can be allowed her opinion, but I myself grow weary of the overwhelming glut of legislation already hanging about our necks. I merely cite Ms. Levine as an example of something less than "thoughtful," glibly abandoning what I see as the Editor's particular role of understanding things of this sort in their complexity rather than in such simple, jejune terms.

Do forgive the tangents; I am not, after all, writing as an Editor, but more like a zebra.

THANKS, SIR FRANCIS, BUT NO THANKS

I was looking at our cat's tail the other day and was struck by its beauty and irrelevance.

Dewey, named after the surgeon who put in my titanium hips, was given to me during my convalescence. He is a white Maine Coon with marvelously long and silky fur and an extraordinary tail. I have often admired his tail's beauty but only now, on the other hand, have I been particularly smitten by its "irrelevance."

What is Dewey doing with this tail anyway? Certainly it has no prehensile function. Even though one may acknowledge that when balancing on the back of a chair his tail may serve the subtle and exquisite function of a gyroscope, I think he could get along perfectly well without it: regard the Manx, poor tailless creature, lovable though it may be. The main use that Dewey contrives for his tail is the brushing clean of tabletops laden with delicate objects and even books, so long as they are good, noisy, crashing-down pieces, preferably photographs in glass frames. Content with the mischief, and having proved the point of gravity, he stretches out and sends further flying whatever artifacts are left (why not a lamp?) to put QED to the Newtonian theorem. Far from making him more fit to survive, his tail, quite to the contrary, for a second or so renders his life in rather dubious balance.

In the wild, wet, Darwinian (or even domestic) jungle, I therefore contend that a cat's tail is of no particular value. What, therefore, is it doing attached to his nether quarters?

And why don't we humans possess one? I have myself certainly done some "balancing acts" in my time and knocked a few artifacts to the floor, particularly once when for a couple of months (long, long, ago) I more or less juggled two girlfriends at the same time, fool that I was. If a tail can help you balance on a real tightrope, it would have done me no good on that one. As a matter of fact, had I had a tail in those days it would have been a dead giveaway. Even with the appendages I possess, I can scarcely get away with any fib whatsoever, and as everyone knows, two girlfriends at once invariably demand of those thus afflicted a real adeptness for persiflage and prevarication. To my *extreme* embarrassment, I was pretty quickly caught out in my machinations, due to the fact that I could hardly keep my hair from standing on end, rolling my eyes, hanging my head, and turning my ears bright pink. If I had had a tail, I would have never lasted two days, much less two months.

I do think, on the other hand, that if we humans had tails their possession would make us both better and worse as a species. We would be "better" because our tail would not allow us such a glib ability to lie, cheat, or practice politics or the law after the fashion we have become so flagrantly accepting of. The tail, its every subtle motion and gesture, would be a dead giveaway.

I can see President Bill commenting about this and that, affirming that he had never had sex with this woman, for example, and particularly THAT one, while all of us watch his tail on television. We would see it waving violently, or quivering hopelessly with some life of its own that even the most accomplished politician would never be able to control, try though he or she might to keep his or her tail in place, calm, poised, and honest.

We would learn every subtle nuance of a tail's motion, and pundits— commenting on how the President or his wife "carried their tails"—would have much, very much indeed, to read into the angle of that appendage, and whether the tip moved ever so slightly when lies were solemnly uttered. Lawyers would discover that lying in court would be much more difficult if they had to deal with a tail sticking out from between the vents, single of course, of their three-piece suits.

If a tail would thus serve humanity positively, acting as a kind of built-in lie detector, I fear it would also cause a great deal of mischief. It is hard enough for the human race to deal with being just a very few different colors without superimposing upon that basically trivial circumstance the problems we would encounter had we tails. The fluffy tails and the long tails, the skinny tails and the short, with an infinitude of nuance between, would immediately demand value judgments about tails, categorizing them as more or less desirable. Society, already stressed by differences in religious, political and color discrepancies, would be rendered all the more inflamed by prejudices against this or that tail-type. Cats are quite above this concern, but we most certainly could not resist it.

This gets me to Sir Frances Crick and his book, *The Astonishing Hypothesis: The Scientific Search for the Soul.* Since unraveling the double helix with Dr. Watson, Crick has concerned his career with demonstrating how our soul, our "vital spirit," "higher purpose" even, possibly is defined by nothing more than a physical sequence of amino acids. Well, that may be true; but I am going to suspect that there is always more to life, the universe, and even ourselves than we can ever truly know. Perhaps I delude myself as I cling to a last, medieval vestige that chooses to believe there is a dash of "magic" about us, somehow or other tucked down between the helices of the DNA molecule.

In the last 500 years we have been reduced from being just a little lower than the angels, at the veritable center of the universe, to nothing more than a sequence of four organic acids, and I'm tired of being pushed around by people making names for themselves. Our humanity becomes as "irrelevant" as a cat's tail. In spite of everything, I am going to affirm that Dewey's tail has a bit of magic in it, defining him as a wondrous creature who, for inexplicable reasons I hope will forever remain inexplicable, is proof against the cold calculations of a narrow-minded science, which assays merely a sequence of wretched chemicals. So, too, will I continue to believe that our soul, angel-winged, lives on, tucked "irrelevantly" away in a deep place beyond the probes of Dr. Crick.

Besides, if we must render ourselves reduced to the absurd—a bunch of chemicals in sequence—I want to ask Dr. Crick what happened to that whole sequence of them that would have given us tails? Why didn't protoman, and protowoman too, have at least some stumpy little appendage? That it would wither away over time, as we became socially and politically organized, might make sense, of course; for under such circumstance anything so apt to be so honest, and give away accordingly our most ulterior motives, would have to be selected out by Darwinian mechanisms.

But, there is simply more to it than Dr. Crick makes out. There is, I shall continue to believe, mystery yet in the cat's tail and equal magic in our lack of one.

And if Dr. Crick deserves a weightier rebuttal to his "Astonishing Hypothesis" relating us, on the great scale of Being, more closely to computers than to angels, I refer him to the comment of a fellow Nobel laureate, Niels Bohr, who quite neatly noted that "a great truth is a truth whose opposite is also a great truth."

So thank you, Sir Francis, but I think not, thanks.

BLESS THE TRIVIA, THAT IT MAY BE DISCARDED

I was cleaning out my desk drawer the other day and noted to myself that the drawer was just like "life."

Who am I, of course, to know just what life is like? I have, for instance, absolutely no idea what a paramecium considers life to be, nor for that matter even the domestic roach, with whom I live in close company, if not quite tooth to jowl. I have some vague feelings of insightfulness regarding the life of the squirrels in our back yard, but that may be a matter of simple anthropomorphizing. Our next-door neighbors, who have a 10-year-old daughter, are a little more "just like us" because our daughter is 11. But they have only one cat, while we have three dogs and three cats, so I would probably miss it with them too. Accordingly, for me to tell them, or anyone, that life is just like my drawer is more presumptuous than I can allow.

In any case, I was cleaning out my desk drawer the other day, something I have not done for at least 10 years, maybe more. Consequently it was stuffed full of sundry impedimenta, including an old dead roach—but no squirrel, plus other ancient debris placed there in the dim past as vitally worth saving. That drawer, I am sure, had rapidly become filled, and I scarcely ever opened it again for fear that something, an 11-year-old for example, might leap forth and grab me by the throat. Somehow I lived out of other drawers, also full, or got along by paying attention only to those things that were actually on top of my desk. Of course you probably pile your desk up too, but because this is in clear view it gets embarrassing if you don't tidy it up every now and then, throwing away 85% of everything you discover, and stacking the journals elsewhere.

The point is that even the most modest, the most subdued of us, live life to the hilt. I gasp as I regard our delightful nurse Mary, who has six horses constantly requiring forkfuls of hay, two boys who always are having to be carted off to play football, baseball, and soccer all at once, every moment of the day, added on to which is merely her husband and a washing machine in ceaseless operation.

It is natural, I mean, to live life to the brim, even if all we do is go back and forth on a well-trodden path twixt home and office. My brain is full, like my drawers, mostly with trivia that easily could be swept out and discarded. Never mind that I am fully aware of the fact that, indeed, if I do sweep something out, leaving for the moment a bit of space, I will very rapidly fill it up again with some other figment of greater or lesser inconsequence.

I count the fact that I can say as much, or so little, as a rather major blessing. After all, most of my mental content is, relatively speaking, trivia.

On the other hand, allow me to contemplate a couple of nasty automobile accidents with which I have been involved, albeit peripherally, in the past two months. One involved a nice family driving down from Ohio to visit relatives in Florida. Their car flew off the road in the wee hours of the night, when the mother, who was driving, fell asleep at the wheel. She is left a quadriplegic, not only to fill her life and mind pondering that most difficult of all circumstances, but also the fact that in that split second when she lost control it cost the life of her husband and badly scarred her daughter's face. The other pertains to a gentleman with a high-powered car to be sold the next day. On a trivial errand he and his little son took the machine out for a last fling late that last night and hit a tree. Tragically, his son remains in a coma, and the father is suffering the mending of numerous broken bones.

One cannot help but think of this lady and this gentleman, good people, who in the lapse of a split second are left for the rest of their lives with a large part of their minds filled with grievance, tragedy, and a relentless guilt which may never be capable of absolution. There, indeed, is a circumstance not readily washed away, cleaned out, or emptied forth from the brain as I did my desk drawer.

If all our minds are stuffed to the brim, there is certainly a great qualitative difference in the stuffing. We can sympathize, maybe are capable of empathy, but, as the old Indian said, we can know nothing until we have walked in the other fellow's moccasins; yet it is hard to walk in moccasins worn by others. How little we can truly know of the hugeness of another's grief or the greatness of their joy, except by guessing at it through our own responses, extrapolating from ourselves as best we can. My own mind, however, is stopped in its tracks way before I reach a point of being able to fathom the depths of feeling of these two automobile drivers. I picture their minds flooded with thoughts beyond my ability to conjure. I put them in the category of those emaciated victims of the holocaust, whose pictures one can hardly look at, but whose souls have truly been seared in ways beyond my little imagining.

So I take heart that the drawer I have cleaned out was filled with nothing but trivial fragments. Soon it will be full again, and I hope with nothing more than other bits of inconsequencia. God spare me the burdens of greater issues.

Like my drawer, I am now cleaning out my brain a bit, thankful that I have that option. I have quit watching all news programs, most TV, and scarcely listen to NPR unless caught in a traffic jam. I did not follow the O. J. Simpson case except by osmosis; ditto the Lewinsky affair. Nor am I going to think much about nuclear blackmail. Perhaps I will write another letter to our congressman about health care, but that will then be that. I am going to shoot for less clutter.

I plan to use the energies thus saved for admiring our cat, conversing with my wife, planting something in the garden (Candide-like), and maybe every now and then even (good grief can one believe it?) stopping to smell the roses if I stumble upon one.

It all comes from simply having cleaned out that drawer, which is still pretty tidy if I do say so myself.

But can it last?

STILL LOOKING GOOD!

In the last week or so I have been compelled to consider my physiognomy.

Such an exercise contains its own peculiar challenges. Generally it is my judgment, professionally as a plastic surgeon and personally as a Human Bean, (as Roald Dahl calls us in *The BFG*) that one should exercise a degree of circumspection in such studies. Happily I am usually too busy to procure much time to look at myself unless I get a zit; even in the morning when I shave I invariably do so in the shower because I like to see if I can perform that surgery blindfolded by steam without nicking myself. As an aside, the best, if somewhat slower, way to perform this function and avoid great gashes is to use a very dull razor. This works well, and the extra time I waste shaving is gained in practicing my Italian; memorized passages of Dante sounding particularly good in high humidity.

In any case, with respect to looking at oneself, I think it best to employ a certain degree of detachment or (to practice my Italian) what in Italy they call *sprezzatura*. I am not absolutely sure what this term means but translate it as having to do with "nonchalance in the face of death," or perhaps, modernizing the image, a liability suit. But yes, that's what I'm seeking as I look in the mirror . . . a dash of nonchalance in the face of death and gravity which, when you get to be 62, you begin to see serious implications relative to . . . .

I have come to this phase of facing my physiognomy as a result of the fact that we have just recently sent forth our last office brochure. This item is one of those usual two-fold bits of heavy paper with a little map on the back showing where our office is. It includes as a bonus a pleasant little drawing of the office itself, complete with a pleasant little cat walking in front of the picket fence, its tail adjusted by my own hand to give it the right angle which, as everyone knows who deals with cats, is crucial in the revelation of feline feelings, whether a 'fraidy, a mad, or a glad cat.

In this brochure, if I may dignify it with such a name, is a picture of my handsome office. There is, also, a bit of a picture of myself to demonstrate that plastic surgeons are fully Human Beans. I am smiling, looking firm about the jawline (or as firm as I pretty much have ever looked), bright of eye, and neither long of earlobe nor droopy of eyelid. There is no trace of laxity beneath the chin and neck area, nary a hint of platysma[1] showing, and my nasolabials and so on look quite fresh. The photograph even then was probably kind, but more noteworthily was taken 10 years ago when I was a hale, hearty, vigorous plastic surgeon, ready to take on a demure challenge and capable, perhaps, even of swinging through the trees.

Well, it is amazing what a few years will do to one, even without having been sued.

---

[1]The platysma, a nasty muscle which lies just beneath, and is attached to, the skin of the face and neck. In the horse it covers the entire body beneath the skin, conveniently allowing the horse, when attacked by a biting fly, to give a shake at the precise point of biting, thus shooing the fly. We humans, having lost this useful capacity, have made up for it by refining to the highest and most subtle degree an ability to manipulate our facial skins, as for example in what the actor Jim Carrey makes millions doing. Then, of course, there is Nicholas Cage, who seems scarcely to have any capacity to move a facial muscle whatsoever, which is what makes him so weirdly compelling. Most of us fall somewhere in between these poles, and our humanity is in some large manner defined by the flicker of our emotions as we let them show in our facial expressions.

Beneath the jaw, however, the platysma muscle, as it peters out at the base of the neck, becomes not only worthless in terms of expressing anything whatsoever, but worse. With time and circumstance it frays and splits, endowing us with those tell-tale bands seen mostly near the midline of the neck, and which so rudely proclaim our antiquity. Seek ye then the yellow pages for your good, old-fashioned, family plastic surgeon, get your platysmas fixed, and (as Dylan Thomas taught us) "go not gently into that good night, but rage, rage, against the dying of the light." And so on and so forth.

In any case, if we are to continue to send out brochures we must therefore have a whole batch printed, and necessarily new pictures fabricated of all of us including myself. I have just finished looking at the proofs, a little wistfully. Indeed, as I did so an involuntary frisson, maybe a perceptible shudder, commanded my nervous system, and only in the nick of time before audibly groaning was I able to beat it back with a dash of *sprezzatura*. For lo, there I am looking ever so slightly, no, perhaps more than ever so slightly, like some kind of old coot. How gray one's hair does get! Mine, as well, I see was in need of cutting, and at this length in the photo I suddenly think I remind myself of George Washington's mother. On the other hand, however, there is at least hair there! I am glad our brochure is not compelled to include a total body x-ray image, however, showing my utter absence of femoral heads and a pile of hardware around the hip joint.

I look closer, clinging to my *sprezzatura* and now see nasty platysmal bands extending sort of from the chin down towards the clavicle, somewhat subtle, but for sure there, causing one to look like an old not-even-coot but a cooter. It is after all those neck bands that make all turtles look old. On the other hand my nasolabial folds still just pass photographically, if the light is good. But what is that? I see a touch of jowl obliterating what was once that terribly firm jawline, a jawline to give any patient the utmost confidence in my ability to, well, perform cardiac resuscitation or maybe bite a tumor. Well, so what? Throw in some more *sprezzatura*, or even salsa, if you please. Actually I never had much of a jawline anyway, especially from the side, but I did ooch by without having to have a chin implant.

In spite of the above, we have got to do this brochure, and a picture of me is going in it. Perhaps I should have rushed over to one of my colleagues in Tallahassee and had some emergency "touch-ups," as they say, but it is too late now.

But hold on, why have expensive surgery when a little photographic retouching may do, or even a little adjustment of the light, like they do in those "Glamour photos"? In any case, I have looked at the proofs and made my choice.

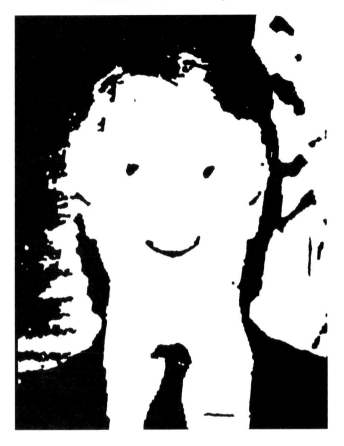

I thought you might like to see it. It is the kind of picture that I think would give a patient a certain degree of confidence in his or her surgeon. What attracted me to this image was the fact that, if just a tiny bit overexposed, it nicely shows up my bright, teddy-bear, button eyes. I like this; all of us have had a teddy bear in our past, and it is comforting to relate that look to your surgeon, surely! Of course, it is nice to have lips, mine having been pretty much washed out, but with the clever assistance of the photographer's retouching pencil we have compensated for that flaw, no worse than Elizabeth Taylor used to do whenever she was on the cover of a magazine in the check-out line of the grocery store. I mean, if she can do it, why can't I? I thought something rather pleasant, as I told the retoucher, something that would be fetching, something looking more like a hospitable ambiance than a hospital ambulance. Why not draw in a nice smile?

So here is the picture. I thought I would run it through here as a final test, knowing that the readers of *The Good, The Bad, and The Homely* have to be discriminating and that you might give me some feedback on how handsome I look. For an old coot.

Anyway, surely there might always be someone out there who would actually prefer their surgeon to look like George Washington's mom!

THE BEST TOAST

I am held in thrall, never mind by our dogs and cats and the terrible guinea pig, by technology.

Oh that I should be a "Noble Savage" (please emphasize Noble) or perhaps live in a "bee-loud glade," etc., in "a cottage of clay and wattles made!" Pure fantasy, of course, because if I were really any kind of "savage" whatsoever I would not even know how to strike a fire, would be allergic to bee stings, and would not recognize a "wattle" if I fell over one.

Although I might formally deny it, I would probably be among the first to beg for a return of my cellular phone, and would certainly plead, as noted in a previous essay, for the instant return of air conditioning, supermarkets, and antibiotics.

The art of living for most of us is necessarily defined in fair measure by what we hope is a decent balance between our computers and a simple fire in the hearth; between the Microsoft Man and Henry David Thoreau; between enormously expensive apparati and contemplation of clouds.

I have struggled vaguely to maintain some reasonable balance within this spectrum at home and in the office, but there is a constant seesawing, and technology, like junk food, is extremely tempting. About three years ago, we took an enormous step for mankind by turning off the television altogether, not being in the least capable, as John Rosemond has advised us in his columns, of sitting down rationally on a weekly basis and choosing which TV programs we and our then nine-year-old daughter might see. TV technology always ooched her away from wholesome programs about, for example, seals or giraffes, towards maybe, for heaven's sake, MTV. There was a constant background racket, inconducive to good digestion, so in a fine little fit one day we turned it off entirely, and, lo, hearth and home were restored. Miss M very pleasantly took to playing with dolls on the floor again, and we read aloud, and so on, marching hand in hand upwards through green pastures into a happy, wholesome future, rather like in "The Sound of Music." I was thrilled, recently, when Miss M actually pointed out to me an assortment of beautiful clouds with a light shining through them "like God." I wanted to exclaim, but did not know the Latin for it, "*ex virtute humanitas.*"

I could cite other, similar examples. The point is that we must not only embrace, but simultaneously actively resist, technology.

On the other hand how can you, quite?

A good friend of mine woke up the other day with a pain in his epigastrium and was so horrified that his wife rushed him to the emergency room. In two days he ended up having a huge mess of tests, including CT scans and cardiac catheterization, all of which ended up negative. Of course, having gone through something like that, it is very nice to possess the information that you not only survived the tests, but that all of your coronaries, your livers, your gallbladders, and your epigastrics are fine and dandy. He got well on his own, but technology must be used because, like Mount Everest, it is there.

A month ago I had a patient who had bumped her breasts and thought she had maybe ruptured her implants, in happier days almost considered high-tech devices themselves. Naturally, I wrung my hands and, being unable to palpate anything of significance, ordered a mammogram. Well, she is, one mammogram and two sonograms later, as well as an inconclusive MRI, now contemplating a gallium scan, because on one of these tests, the implants apparently being hale and hearty, a tiny spot was seen. This is probably a very small cyst, but had to be worked up in full technological fashion nevertheless. As I discussed her case with the radiologist, the delightful Dr.

Mary Swain, she wrung her hands a bit too, allowing that in her specialty the radiologist tries very hard to focus essentially on questions at hand, hoping that nothing else will come up that requires expensive batteries of further elaborate tests. But if it does, technology and costs are for sure waiting in the wings. Better that, however, than living in the "hut of clay and wattles made," with fleas, and a cancer lurking in your bosom.

Although less than many physicians and some of you, even I battle with technological questions. Although good, old-fashioned, small-town family plastic surgery is really a rather low-tech specialty (you can take a skin graft with a razor blade after all) I am still confounded in my response to patients regarding their spider veins and dermal varicosities. In highly low-tech fashion, I inject these with 23% saline solution, which seems to me to work right well. It is also extremely cheap. It is rather fun to do, too. We have psychiatrists up here who do it, and "vein clinics" too, which shows you how much fun it's got to be. But my patients are more and more asking me about using a laser on those tiny spots. They ask "if the laser works better."

I have no idea if the laser works better. I don't, however, think it is "magic" either. But I do tell patients that I think it's an awful lot more expensive, because whoever is going to be lasering you is probably going to be looking to you also to help pay for the fairly expensive machinery and maybe even a Park Avenue address. My patients, though placated, are still slightly suspicious, for we are trained to consider all that is glitz gold, and laser now has about it an entire cachet of wonder, augmented by those schemes to use it to shoot down enemy ballistic missiles somewhere out near the heliosphere. If it can do that, it should certainly get rid of spider veins quite miraculously.

But, thank heavens, patients in the majority still have a lot of common sense about these issues, so it all works out fine, especially if you give them a low-tech smile.

Nevertheless, even I wonder if the laser works better. Does anyone really know? This very morning I am going to be injecting someone's veins.

I will probably put on my 2.5x loupes, which will be the nearest thing to high tech I'm going to apply to this matter. I have made my stand, I think. If people want to go to someone who uses a laser on them, they certainly may but as for me, when I finish with this case, I'm going to rush to the kitchen and make myself a toasted peanut butter and jelly sandwich. I consider this a very low-tech sandwich.

Yet, I know that one of these days I will be tempted when I see in *The Sharper Image* catalog to buy after all a "Laser Toaster" or in Hammacher-Schlemmer "the Best Laser Toaster."

For the present, however, I am going to do my best to resist getting one. They say, after all, the best toast is made with a fork over a peat fire.

Which causes me to wonder about faggots? Or maybe even wattles?

MODEM UPGRADE

Why I, who just last month was stopping barely short of the notion of living in "a hut of clay and wattles made," should have a computer at all still remains rather beyond me. As you now know, my office is a small cottage surrounded by a picket fence and embraced by a couple of large live oaks, neither of which is very high-tech. For years we got along very well with the ordinary and usual appointment book, which I knew perfectly well how to flip through when I sought permission to have lunch with someone. I think it was when the roof took to leaking and our walls rotted out as a result of moisture wicking up by way of confederate jasmine growing within them, that we entered the modern era. We got plastic walls and a computer.

In any case, I remember thinking, if we are to have plastic siding, why not do something further flashy. Other great centers were all computerized, especially the dermatologist's, and I thought vaguely that getting a computer might lessen the chores of what I shall hazard to call my "clerical staff," who were up to this point sitting on the equivalent of high stools, filling out onslaughts of forms armed only with bottles of ink and a quill. We got the computer and now get to spend a good deal of interesting time figuring out "what is wrong with it?" and, when nothing is, gathering around it breathlessly to consult it as though it were an oracle ensconced on a tripod.

All of us, by some kind of osmotic process, have now learned just barely enough about which keys to push in which sequence to get whatever. "Escape-Escape" is the key key. Now, in the veritable grip of technology, we press on. Of course, we also got a fax machine, and I became a wanton, faxing fool.

Then we got something further called "Déjà Vu," which by its ability to converse with AIX, our basis system, allows us to hook up to our domestic modems standing by our, so to speak, homely hearths at home. To look at my little office building from outside you would never guess how much wire winds hither and yonder within, and just to get out of the place at night now requires the pursuit of a fairly elaborate algorithm to make sure "this" is off, "this" is on, "that" unplugged, and "that there" plugged.

I did not, after all, choose to become a surgeon—perhaps I should say a plastic surgeon so as not to offend other surgeons—in order to be a computer technician. As a matter of fact, I chose surgery, particularly perhaps plastic surgery, in no small measure because it seemed on the whole a pretty low-tech specialty.

Sutures, for example, have been around for quite a few thousand years and somehow or other I like the sound of that. Sometimes I quite consciously feel a curious (small) elation over the fact, as I put in a bit of suture somewhere, that I am using a technique employed effectively at least 5000 years ago by the Egyptian embalmers, who were sort of prototype, albeit postmortem, plastic surgeons. Like eye makeup for ladies, some things have simply been around since time immemorial because they work, and one can maybe take a bit of pleasure in the fact. Even skin staples are nothing more than a somewhat more convenient substitute for a well-endowed beetle, the latter being hard to store, and the art of just how much pressure to exert on their thorax to make them approximate their mandibles lost in the mists of history.

My office, in any case, is all hooked up now, poised, if not fully ready, to enter the great world of communications, Internet, and the World Wide Web. We had some frustrating moments when we replaced our modems and put in Déjà Vu: Our man who installed our upgrade is an earnest, no-nonsense person, as you would expect from someone who plays the bagpipe and arrived en route to a practice session fully kilted and dirked. There was a lot of trouble with my keyboard at home when, for mysterious reasons, the "F" and "Enter" keys utterly changed identity. It took awhile to trace it to Dewey, our cat, who had apparently jumped on the wrong set of keys, thinking he was writing a sonnet but in fact remapping a variety of functions. You would have thought with all this technology that someone would have built into the system an anti-cat protection device.

But never mind that. Now, from the comforts of my own kitchen at home, over a glass of milk and a jalapeño pepper, I can access patients' addresses and telephone numbers by hotline to my office. This is, however, only a small part of what I am further aspiring towards. Heady with the thrill of all these marvels, I am secretly putting myself in the mode of practicing surgery from a distance.

About a month ago I was reading about "Scientist Ian Hunter," a denizen of M.I.T., who even now has devised the technology, if you have a modem and a bit of a robot, so that you, the great surgeon in Tallahassee, or Fort Lauderdale, or Singapore, may operate on a patient supine in Los Angeles. Not that I would ever want to operate on anyone in Los Angeles, God forbid! It is the principle that is beguiling.

Pretty soon, as I see it from our kitchen, over a leisurely second cup of morning coffee, we surgeons will be able to click on the little "Surgery" icon, don a pair of comfortable old gloves wired to our modem, and with "virtual vision" through the eyes of the remote robot, command that interesting presence to perfectly duplicate every twitch and twiddle of our fingers. Such "slave surgeons," whom I picture looming over the patient like one of those Darleks out of *Doctor Who*, will be tirelessly on duty 24 hours a day at our beck and whim. If over a third cup of coffee we want to operate on our patient who is vacationing in Mongolia, and who has maybe ruptured his/her appendix, all we will need to know is the Mongolian country code; thus, from the veritable comfort of our home, our own cat handy, we will be able to fully fulfill our ancient surgical function.

Of course, they may not have a proper robot in Ulan Bator. It is one of the inconveniences of high technology that you have to have it to use it.

The patient, of course, would then have to get in touch with the local Mongolian Medical Society, as I always instruct my patients to do in case of need, to find a local Mongolian surgeon. He (I am not sure yet if "she" exists over there) would then have to drag himself from his home—just possibly a "hut of clay and wattles made"—possibly grumpy over being called away from his warm fire and his cat.

You know how those Mongolian surgeons are!

Or am I speaking of myself?

Surely not!

[STAYING LOOSE]

I n a fast changing world, more specifically the fast changing world
of "modern medicine," one has to learn to be "flexible."

I am trying, within grave restrictions, to do so.

This may be harder for me than it is for the rest of you, who may be
born naturally flexible. I wasn't. I have always had extremely stiff joints. For
a long time, I thought it was just a dash of fibrosis about the bursae, and I
limped along right well through life, quite content. Then some radiology
technician watching me limp along suggested (he had an idle moment) that
he shoot a shot of my joints, for sport. I had an idle moment before a surgery case, so said "why not? What's a few Röntgens to someone who is getting on to being an old coot?"

The rest was history, as they say. The next thing I knew the formidable
Dr. Dewey, orthopod extraordinaire, had me on an operating room table
replacing both my hip joints. As a result I am a little bit more flexible: But
what about my shoulders? What about my brain?

This flexibility thing is hard too because of habit. On the whole, I like to
learn something, and to think that once I've learned it, it will never change.
I am quite content that it should not. If it works, why go fooling around
looking for something else that works? Not to say I totally deny the hope of
progress: I would, after all, much rather fly the Atlantic in a jumbo jet than
in the Spirit of St. Louis.

But surely some things can be left alone, and if not, why not?

I bring this all up as it applies to medicine because of a difficult point encountered at a recent Quality Assurance Committee meeting on which I diffidently serve. I am pleased to be on this committee even though I am not sure I know how to spell assurence (sic). All sorts of arcane matters are discussed, with heavy breathing and a lot of sighs on the part of the participants. Some of us know not much about what is going on, but others of us, like the formidable Matt Cohen, MD, know everything about what is going on, and somehow point us more or less into the future.

But the interesting and quite audible sigh I heard at the last meeting had to do with a government point. In its wisdom, the aforesaid government is mandating a certain number of forms that must be on all patients' office records, and if not there the doctor will be tortured. Even (good grief!) specialists will now have to toe the line and make a show of using these checklists. One point on a form all to itself documents that we have asked patients if they have a "living will." The question is slightly awkward when you are discussing forthcoming surgery, let us say the removal of a wart or release of a trigger finger, with a brand new patient. There is a "yes" box, which you get to check in the way of compensation. It is the kind of question that we will now have to learn to ask merrily, and in good humor, with a big smile. Then, of course, there is a great new version of the great old checklist for the pediatricians regarding children's immunizations.

It was interesting to me to see with what subtlety this updated device, being a government form, precipitates confusion and irritation, e.g., in fact, for example, that whoever has contrived it decided, in wanting to make his or her dubious mark within the great bureaucracy of form design, that the DPT immunization should no longer be identified by this hallowed abbreviation, known forever to us all, but is now to be called the DTP. It is the indiscriminate taking of such liberties that galls.

Who, and under what authority, has decided to put the T between the D and the P rather than where it ought to be at the end of the D and P? It is simply incomprehensible to me that anyone should be so rude, and to what purpose? Why? Who makes these decisions? Besides, it seems to me so vastly more euphonious to say "DPT" as opposed to "DTP." I have, as you see, taken severe umbrage and so, I thought, did the entire committee (with the exception of our chief, Dr. William Price, who has become hardened) to this molestation of ancient abbreviations.

Well, the new age continues to dawn for sure. So, trying to be flexible, I have been practicing saying, trippingly on the tongue, "DTP," in case I meet with some federal overseer. I have become quite good at it. I'm almost as good at it as when I used to say "DPT."

My fear, now, is that I may grow perversely fond even of DTP.

It takes a little practice, but if I can make the switch so can you. Try saying it to yourself a few times. I would be happy to hear from you regarding your preference, and will even reply with a real, not a form, letter.

In any case, you see, I find myself yet capable of a just sufficient degree of residual flexibility. Even my hips are moving a little better lately, I think. But that may just be a rise in the barometric pressure.

KEEPING
THE BALANCE

I recently had a vaguely disturbing insight into my life's evolving circumstance.

It was on Thanksgiving weekend and, having given due thanks, truly, and having enjoyed the abundant delicacies of the table and its bird, and being surrounded by good cheer among family and two or three friends, I then fell by Saturday evening into what my wife calls a "generic depression."

I do not think, honestly, I am afflicted by any bipolarity, and on the whole feel rather even-tempered, content, and brightly disposed. Occasionally, however, I perceive myself, when the wind is south–southeast and the barometric pressure falling, as being affected by elemental forces emanating more from the spleen, or perhaps the liver, than the brain. I hope in such instances to o'erleap myself, and as a restorative do something more or less positive. If that fails, I will look at our cats and marvel in their excellence, a much-to-be preferred expedient compared to making a run for junk food, well recognized by all authorities as a great depressant in themselves.

Thanksgiving Day we had been busy, buffing the house so it looked half-presentable to our guests; my wife labored over her Cuisinart; I turned on the air-conditioning and built a cheery fire. Our guests arrived. Grace at the bountiful table went badly, I thought. Our daughter, home from college, claims to be a great atheist; our younger daughter believes in a Being greater than herself, I think, but her forms of saying Thanks at the table are highly complex, more reminiscent of a mass in Saint Peters than anything our company could easily bear. Our guests themselves were a motley crew: one professes world-weariness and cynicism; another is such a merry spirit that God seems almost irrelevant in his universe; and, finally, an unknown quantity partook with us, an English lady, an archivist at a great museum in London, therefore surely idiosyncratic, and who we accordingly knew not how to handle whatsoever.

I am off on a tangent, however; suffice it that my wife brightly suggested we all give our own silent thanks, like children are supposed to do in schools. The suggestion sounded a decent solution in contradistinction to my intoning some awkward platitude. Silence, however, didn't work particularly well either. When everyone is saying "silent thanks," how do you know when everyone else is finished? We all pretty dutifully bowed our heads, but as I lifted mine slightly upwards, to peek, I saw that almost everyone else at the table was peeking too, signifying to me that everyone was far more preoccupied by finding out their status within the scheme of this exercise, with peeking, rather than with thanksgiving. We all ended up smiling more or less gently at one another, while our youngest daughter, Meredith, finished crossing herself and making various passes in the air.

We laid to. We had a hearty time. The next day we rested from our exertions, giving grateful thanks that the house was more or less restored to a semblance of home. The cats came out from their hiding places. The dogs roamed free once again. We ate leftovers, and were pleased.

But by Saturday a windshift brought with it this nagging bit of "generic depression." I searched restlessly for something to be genuinely depressed over, but was thwarted at every turn. Well, how about my age? When one is over three score that can usually be brought to bear; but my circulatory system is pretty good, I am HIV negative, and my prostate apparently feels very nice to my physician, who says it is only a tiny bit enlarged.

Money. That is often a good reason to be depressed. Yes, I've lost a goodly little deal in an investment, and probably will lose more. But somehow or other we still seem to be living perfectly comfortably, and this year we have assimilated a new roof, a new air-conditioner upstairs, and a refurbishment of what I shall hopefully call our garden. True, it would be nice if I were in some lovely financial position where I could retire before I am 85, but really, one must ask oneself, why cavil?

People get depressed, I guess, over sex sometimes. Well, forgive me for not going into any details, but I am simply not depressed over sex.

I spent both Saturday and Sunday sort of moping about. I plucked at the piano ever so slightly but nothing sounded quite right. I dug in desultory fashion in the garden a wee bit, but it was not particularly satisfying. I read fitfully and looked at a book of paintings, finding them slightly bland. I had a peanut butter and jelly sandwich and a glass of cold milk, neither of which I consider "junk food," but my spirit was only uplifted for the 30 seconds it took to eat these devisings.

Then came Monday. It was a struggle more or less to get up and I would have rather not. I arose, nonetheless, as we good physicians must. I showered. I put on one sock, then the other. I went to the office.

Astonishingly I was suddenly cured, cured and a little horrified all at once.

We had a pleasant, vigorous day at the office. Everyone was in good spirits and had had a wonderful Thanksgiving holiday. I have a delightful office staff, and we all rushed about merrily helping each other out. Many patients shared with us dashes of gossip about this and that going on in town. My bit of surgery went beautifully. The music was excellent, a combination of "Out of Africa" on one cassette and Enya on another. Patients were pleased, and complimented my staff and myself on a number of pleasant little occasions. I paid them nice compliments in return.

So also went Tuesday and Wednesday. I am led to think how good it is to have the work all of us do. And yet, I shudder to think, I hope not, but just conceivably, that I have entered insidiously into that terrible circumstance where too much a proportion of one's happiness is found in one's work. Could this be true? Will it get worse? Must decent work become so gratifying that it absorbs one? I have had a glimpse of how it can happen, and with good reason, too.

One must be on guard, perhaps, and not forget the joys of looking at one's cats, or of reading one's wife a bit of a poem every now and then.

A little Ogden Nash, at least.

ON MOTHERHOOD, INDEED!

Stop, don't read any further if you do not want to hear a male plastic surgeon commenting about childbirth and motherhood. On the other hand, if you could conceive that I have anything whatsoever to guess about this subject, read on. Indeed, you may even read on out of mere morbid curiosity.

Yes, you are entitled to ask why I am writing about such an arcane subject so far removed from both my practice and experience. Well, to be brief, I'm writing it as a small act of defiance, to prove the point that I believe one can, after all and contrary to "reason," still have an opinion about matters utterly beyond one's own intimate experience.

This . . . what shall I call it? . . . "conceit" became manifest to me as a result of a conversation I was having with a charming patient who is also a bit of a friend I admire. She is an English lady in the highest tradition of that doughty breed, rather like that Mrs. Baker who helped her husband explore the upper reaches of the Nile while wearing hoop skirts and voluminous pantaloons. She speaks the Queen's English, and has trailing about her remnants of the glory of Empire and the 11th edition of the *Encyclopaedia Britannica*. If her nose is slightly, and why not say justly, elevated it is offset by a merry twinkle of the eye, a fanciful play at the corners of her mouth, and a cavalier attitude towards life's foibles.

I was visiting her at her home, as she was recovering from a *soupçon* of surgery, and as the morning sun poured in through the French doors ("windows" in England) revealing the charming garden without, we conversed.

"We" comprised herself, her daughter, and one of my various personalities, this one reflecting my interpretation of urbanity, worldliness, Noel Coward, etc. At the very worse, it is good for a laugh.

In any case, we were talking . . . can you believe it here in little old Tallahassee! . . . about Ralph Waldo Emerson. His essay "On Marriage" was broached, to which Mrs. Winters, in a diction impeccably 11th edition (*vide supra*), noted that it was quite ridiculous that he should be writing on marriage when he was never married!

But, after all, he had been madly in love. Distraction over the youthful death of his beloved had driven him from Puritan Massachusetts to his first trip to Europe, landing him in Sicily in 1831, an eye-opening experience. He went on to transcend tragedy and to found the transcendental school of native New England thought. Even if he wasn't "married" surely being madly in love is worth something! "A few choice words on marriage should not be denied a broken heart," I suggested.

Joanne, the attentive daughter, demurred, siding with her mom on the point that if he had never married he could never write about it.

"I have never flown wingless through the air, like Superman, either," I said, "but I know I could write about it. You don't have to experience things to write about them. True, many might think you foolish and ignorant, as they might if I were to write about motherhood and being pregnant; but still I could write about it, couldn't I?"

"Good heavens, no!" sniffed my friend.

"Of course not," echoed her daughter who added "and in any case I would never read it if you did."

Accordingly . . . I want to say precisely this about childbirthing and motherhood: It is an extraordinary experience, which only ladies, with the exception of Arnold Schwarzenegger in the movie "Junior," have ever experienced to my knowledge. Psychologists and sociologists and all sorts of other people have been trying, in the last few decades, to bring us men into the experience far more intimately: and in rather half-hearted fashion we have become half-baked participants in the act of childbirth, and even motherhood. We have come a long way past simply smoking cigarettes out in some corridor while this thing happens. We are there, making gallant attempts at being supportive, and repressing any urges to verbalize on the cost of a college education or the dangers of over-population. We have our pictures taken while holding the baby, all red and waxy, with a little cap on its head. We try with indifferent success not to faint.

As for moms themselves, the experience must be one with sufficient enticements to keep ladies world-wide busy having babies, despite the pitfalls and pain that this sometimes entails. I cannot, of course, speak from direct experience; but there is more to it than simply one's skin glowing with the radiant expectation of motherhood in the offing, or the selfless bearing of a great responsibility and a great act of creation. There is the great Nobility of Motherhood, as an expression of faith in the future, of Hope, of Possibility, and a means of expressing love and giving at its highest level. I think, as a matter of fact, there is a lot that goes into procreation, childbearing, and motherhood that even mothers themselves can hardly describe or quite know the meaning of.

I do not see why in the world I cannot say as much, even though I have never been a mom.

Perhaps, on the other hand and as an actual dad, I can take this moment to say I am grateful to the mothers of this world, particularly the mother of our children, and my own mom.

As a matter of fact, come to think of it, I think I would have more difficulty writing an essay on "fatherhood." Fatherhood I cannot figure out at all. It is most difficult to understand what in the world is the meaning of fatherhood. I do my best as a father but still (metaphorically speaking) have the vague sensation that I am walking around in galoshes, ankle deep in mud. It is beyond my interpretation. I try to be a good father but am overly indulgent probably. When I try to be a disciplinarian I muff it, and everyone laughs. Fatherhood is extremely hard on the ego, and it is almost beyond my interpretation in the essay form.

No, my friends are wrong. Trust me, I feel much more confident writing on something I know nothing about. That way you don't have to be affected by any facts you might happen to possess, which are altogether too confusing.

Stay tuned for my next essay, then, which may be on flying through the air like Superman. Nor will I accept any comments from the scientists among you who, grimly clinging to your facts, might castigate this essay as mere BS.

As I said, you didn't need to read it; but if you did welcome to the club!

THE HOMELY VIEW

I should not be writing this. "Bioethics" is, after all, a very serious business, and a slippery one too. Like Motherhood, it is easier mentioned, particularly by those of us who will never be Mothers, than done. One can always sit around like Aristotle, with a beer in hand and propound on Ethics of any sort, even with a capital "E." And yet I suspect that the more one is absolute about one's pronouncements, the more readily Life can, in its perverse and insidious way, slip into the equation some dumbfounding bit of Tomfoolery that throws those famous best laid plans of men and mice awry.

For what it is worth, my own view is that there is a real place for ethical Generalities, such as "Beauty is Truth and Truth Beauty" and "The Golden Rule" and other such big principles, allowing the specifics, so multitudinous and capable of hair-splitting, to take care of themselves as the circumstance dictates.

But, as I said, I am not sure I know why I am writing about Ethics. The challenge to do so is, of course, intriguing because I am not a philosopher well versed in this topic, but if I have rashly allowed myself a few thoughts on Motherhood, so why not Ethics? In the final analysis (surely you will agree!) there is nothing more important than the ethics for which we stand in doing whatever anyone does, even a President, and therefore we should attempt a gracious tolerance for those who might want, after all, to give ethical values the least passing thought. Doubtless our President has himself, indeed, given the least passing thought to ethical values, or surely not much less than that.

As for myself, as I contemplate the matter, I do not think I have ever in the practice of medicine and surgery dealt in some excruciating fashion with a "Great Ethical Question." Immediately, I think I must be practicing some form of Denial or be incredibly naive; for indeed a case could be made for the fact that every action we take has its own ethic, from which ripples spread out as in those famous ponds into which stones are thrown.

God knows how anyone, myself included, tolerated that pair of weeks during my general surgery residency when I had a bit of what I shall call a "nervous breakdown," and fled rather curiously. That egregious lapse, however, had nothing to do with bioethics other than the fact that I just quit functioning. Well, a point can be derived from even this experience: that one must guard against madmen being one's surgeon, and remember too that madmen are sometimes not so easily identified and may, astonishingly, project their madness all about them, doing strange injury, even onto whole peoples who may, their ethics displaced elsewhere, come to accept mutely the "ethics" of, say, the extermination of a whole race of people. None of us can be fully trusted always to know or be willing to recognize what is right, and stand up for it as well. Remember the townspeople in *High Noon*?

Even so and by all means, we can at least be watchful against some sly madness taking over our ethical values. It has happened, to highly intelligent folks too, if we regard the ravages and distortion that afflicted the Germans in the 1930s.

As for the specific ethics of Life and Death, it may be that there can never be written final words covering every situation. If words, on the other hand, must be written, as we inevitably must try, I think I would prefer them written by a poet, Keats indeed!, than by any committee, particularly political. Was it William of Occam who had the razor, now named after him, who showed that the shaving of circumstance into ever thinner slices left you not so much with knowledge of whatever you are shaving (I picture a turnip) but with nothing? The whole circumstance, the "Tao of

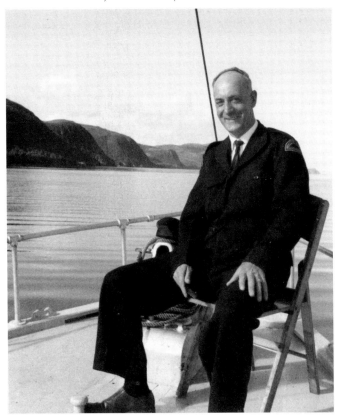

Jack Dowding, cook-crewman on "The Doctor's Boat,"
as good and dear a man as anyone could wish to meet.

Being" as I think they call it, the *unus mundus* of Paracelsus, must never be forgotten.

As for myself, and beyond my "madness" during my surgical residency, up in Newfoundland I did once face a bit of Life and Death served up on the platter of possible ethical inquiry. On this isolated coast, where I had the residents of twelve little fishing villages to care for, accessible only by "the doctor's boat" put at my disposal, I found myself faced with the great ethical question of a little euthanasia. The cook-crewman of the doctor's boat, a forty-foot craft that at 7 knots withstood rough seas fairly well, was a man I much loved and honor to this day. He came down with a cancer of the colon.

At the little cottage hospital four hours away, down the coast and around Connaigre Head, they opened him up, and found widely disseminated metastases. He came home to our little village, worked a little longer after his recovery from the surgery, and then took desperately ill. He refused further surgery, particularly a colostomy, and it being winter and we being fogbound, there was in any case really no way out. His bowel became completely obstructed, and he was living in great pain. I had some IV fluids, and started a drip in his cottage home, his family standing about. Except for the IV, the scene could have been in the mid-19th century as opposed to mid-20th. His pain was intractable. The family, and my friend himself, begged relief. Their meaning was perfectly clear to me. How much morphine did I give him? I have no idea, but he fell, finally, quietly, asleep and died.

I have never known if my dose killed him. If it did, I have not the least feeling of guilt or violation of what I shall call my ethical principles. If I did not, he had a nice sleep and died peacefully in it. Occam, with his razor, could shave that dose down ever so thinly, and yet not know if it was deadly or palliative. I do know that my friend died, surrounded by a loving family in the soft light of the kerosene lamp, for there was no electricity. He was buried in the lovely little churchyard hard by the lovely little Anglican church he had attended all his life, we singing for his soul. Keats could not have had, under that grey sky with snow coming on, better last rites.

But here, of course, is the rub, the fly in my ointment, namely, that what the old fashioned medical practitioner could do, and do let us hope very wisely indeed, we cannot. He (in those days) practiced in an isolation the equivalent of Newfoundland's south coast, unscrutinized by the media and almost by the law, and as well was granted the utmost respect and trust of his patients and their families. We, on the other hand, have our every act recorded and dissected under a microscope. There is no way, accordingly, that we can administer "just a touch" of euthanasia and allow it to be unknown, almost to ourselves, what we have done. Clearly the individual can, under such circumstances, do what no committee can. No "committee" can say "Let us give this dose of morphine. Maybe it will kill him, and maybe it won't." For better or worse, we have not the luxury of equivocation.

Even so, from my Newfoundland experience I came indeed to trust the image of the "old family doctor" who lived among his patients. There are, as any loving people know, understandings that words cannot frame. We can legislate ourselves from here to perdition, write millions of words that are supposed to cover every contingency, and yet will we have compassion? In this world of committees, agencies, and bureaucracies—all of which may certainly be composed of compassionate, caring, and hard-working people—there is little latitude beyond what their rules and words and job descriptions allow. We see it all the time now, when we dial the number of these laudable institutions, and are given a menu of buttons to push, only to be told finally that you must dial another number, or another.

I humbly think it is important that we find a gentle way to keep individual circumstance before us. We cannot go back to Newfoundland and the mid-19th century, nor would we want to, but let me hope, as we are led into the future by lawyers, committees, and Presidents, that jargon will not be made an equivalent of Truth, Beauty, Care, and Compassion.

That, to me, is the challenge to modern Bioethics.

BUT IS IT A SHOE?

I do not mean to accuse myself unfairly, but I vaguely wonder if, as people get older, they begin not so much to trust the "realities" of circumstance?

In college, as a callow youth when I first read of Dr. Johnson's mighty kicking of the stone, and crying out "Thus I refute Berkeley," it seemed to me indeed that "stoniness" and the sore toe combined made a quite patently clear case for materialism.

This business of things being not what they appeared seemed to me altogether superfluous, and it was quite sufficient for my prosaic needs that what seemed so, in fact, was. Our President, of course, has recently led the way otherwise by demonstrating that what seemed so obviously so, in fact, wasn't.

The issue becomes one more of metaphysics, towards which I do not think that Dr. Johnson was very generously disposed. For most of us, however, I think that as we get older and by progressive degrees closer to those "Intimations of Mortality" we become a little more metaphysical. The fact may be demonstrable by what I believe would be the statistically significant preference for older folks to gravitate toward religion, while the young, often enough, have to have it forced down their throats. I do not think the experiment has been done, but I would almost venture to say that if you gave a random population of children and septuagenarians a choice between a lollipop and a sermon that there might well be a meaningful discrepancy in their choices. Not that I am averse to a lollipop myself, and am as capable of judging the excellence of a sermon by its brevity as I was in my youth. In other words, I still have a long way to go in the pursuit of the metaphysical.

Dragging myself back to my primary thesis, however, I rather like to think that the universe may be quite different from what our studies have taught us to think of it as being. What we think we know is derived from the study of a narrow spectrum of facts which we are pleased to study because they are studyable, capable of being examined, categorized, analyzed, and concluded therefrom with all the marvelous majesty of our species. It is difficult to remove ourselves from the rut amounting perhaps to a deep trench that we create for ourselves as we pace back and forth massaging our facts. How, anyway, in the practice of medicine or life itself, can we do more than peruse that narrow spectrum that is our lot to live within? No matter how hard we try, we will never see, like the bee, whatever lurks in the wavelengths of the ultraviolet. Even the mighty brain cannot dream in images beyond those shaped by the forms and formalities of our experience. And after all, living within so thin a perspective, there is sufficiency aplenty for us to marvel at, to be amazed by, to create with, and to turn to what we may hope may be of good use. If the Real Great White Light Bulb of Revelation turned on, we might hardly be able to bear it any more than Dante in the hundredth Canto of the *Divine Comedy*.

As I think thus I am reminded of the story of the great 17th century English antiquary, Sir Robert Cotton. This gentleman of excellent intelligence was one evening, in the domestic comfort of his home "magnifying of a shoe, (to determine whether) it was Moses's or Noah's, and wondering at the strange shape and fashion of it." Entered his good wife, clearly a lady of practical nature and probably a Mom to boot, to remark of the formless lump of clay, "But, Mr. Cotton . . . *are you sure it's a shoe?*" The learned arguments, the recondite subtlety, the finest points as to whether the lump in question belonged to Moses or Noah gave up the ghost before the brilliant illumination of common sense. I like to hope that without more ado Mrs.

Cotton rolled up her sleeves and did the dishes, leaving Sir Robert to his devices and thoughts.

I often think, when I get elaborate . . . particularly with the children . . . that I had at least ought to try and make sure, indeed, 'twere a shoe or not!

Allow me to apply this question to my own medical practice: For example, take this infernal machine, the laser, that is consuming the pop-dermatologist-cum-plastic-surgeon-and-anyone-else-who-wants-to-afford-one. Cheered on by the even more pop media, we are almost forced to ascribe to this modification of the blow-torch a well-nigh magical means of restoring our poor integument. Never mind that there is truth in this, by the way. The point is that we know minute things about the wave length at which vaporization of cells will occur, the number of joules that must be exerted, and the precise time these joules are to be applied. We make a nice distinction, almost as nice as Sir Robert's, to make sure that we know that this instrument does not really burn, but (fine difference!) merely explodes a few skin cells by "vaporization." We happily now have at our disposal, we believe, a much more discrete means, compared to the blow torch, of not providing the patient with a third degree burn to the face. I consider this, naturally, a lucky point in our favor, while not very eagerly awaiting the next phase of the media's enthusiasm, namely, that of reporting on the various wretched disasters that laserizing a patient may be prone to. It is a "chicken point," but in the loneliness of my little solo practice I sometimes catch myself wondering if, by mere accident, I were to provide someone with a nice full thickness burn and nasty scar what then shall I do with all the knowledge I now possess on the physics of high energy light? To be blunt, will the jury be impressed?

Such a pity that I find myself thinking such things! But there is simply more to everything than it seems, by a long shot, and forgive me for being trite to say so.

As for medical care in general, we think we know what it is, but sometimes I wonder. It is a great deal more than even a CT scan, of course. It is a great deal more than what the poor government is trying to define it as being, scrutinize though they may through mighty magnifying lenses vastly more intense and powerful than those of Sir Robert's. Their arguments, like his, are designed to support preconceptions which may be based upon thoroughly false premises, such as, for example, that health care is a "product," and therefore like any product subject to economic theory, leading thereby to the rich possibility that government manipulation can do as much for medical "care" as it is supposed to do for interventions elsewhere.

But never mind the poor government, always a convenient scapegoat. Look to thyself! I swear to attempt it, acknowledging before the fact that even though my own specialty may not lie in making the distinction between whether or not this or that may belong to Moses or Noah, I am quite as capable as Sir Robert of allowing common sense to elude me in order to have it "my way." The goal, after all, is to make out of life what you like, and I can only hope that my presumptions are as innocent as his.

One has to admire Mrs. Cotton. She knew her husband all too well. I think he was lucky to have been married to her. She was probably a very good cook too, washed his socks, and clearly kept him from falling from high places and into gutters.

Meanwhile, I have not yet bought a laser and wring my hands that all my colleagues are going to leave me irretrievably in their dust, destitute. Instead of spending all that money, however, first I want to see if I can determine (my own wife, thank goodness, will be a big help in this endeavor!) whether or not I am really dealing with a shoe.

With lollipops and sermons, on the other hand, I'll take my chances.

END OF THE BEGINNING

My own theory of the brain's functioning is rather simple: *When you are born, that gruel we thereafter call the brain is a pretty watery affair, a kind of primordial alphabet* soup with various letters and syllables, and maybe even a few tentative phrases scattered about in the dark. Between these islands of light course vague dendritic tendrils, which, though real, are as insubstantial as those strange "strings" that theory speculates somehow bind the universe together.

In due course, as I see it, the soup thickens, as things do with a little boiling, and certain patterns of information exchange begin to develop between the flashes of light. Music begins to be heard. Energy becomes channeled, patterns of electric flow are established, and coalescences occur. The brain, firming up like a fine aspic or our universe ten billion years ago, becomes the powerful organ we know and love. It is now capable of almost anything including, if you are born with a direct connection between part A and part B, the ability to come up with the cube root of 1.534×10^7 in a split instant. To do that, in my estimation, takes such a deeply dug trench, or rather such a large-bore, readily conductive pathway between A and B as to amount to a short circuit, leaving the poor idiot-savant thus possessed almost paralyzed when it comes to other, more mundane thought processes.

I also think that some people's brains, and certainly my own, are initially, and not unusually, remain more watery than others, and that the connections between those millions upon billions of points of light are a bit more tenuous. As an aside, and likely enough no more than pure prejudice on my part (laced with envy!) I think that people who can make a lot of money have slightly firmer brains than I who write this and maybe even you who read. (It may be only a further bias of mine, and forgive me because I do not mean to be insulting, but I wonder at the proportion of people with lots and lots of money, or maybe firm brains too, who read any of this.) Although, like any watery adolescent, I am still capable of wearing a Dr. Seuss hat (see page 93), with age, perforce it being thrust upon you, the brain does finally get a little firmer, even if you are not granted greater shrewdness economically.

But with age, alas!, you have been doing the same thing for so long, repeating the same patterns so often, that your electric circuits are pretty much apt to follow those easiest well-worn paths of least resistance, like cows at dusk wending their way homeward to the happy barn by tracks deeply eroded through time and habit.

And so what?

So, it has crossed my mind at age 63 that one of these days I will some-day have to begin to start thinking about—I can scarcely write it—*Retirement*! Yes, conceivably even I, though so "young," with merely a few platysmal bands sagging in my neck. But yet I have no synaptic connections in my brain with any sort of retirement node. It is somewhere lost in the watery darkness, and I suppose I will have to find some path, some devious unused bit of circuitry, to find a way to illuminate that point, even with fee-ble wattage.

I glance on random occasions, but more often in response to a question by a patient, at a wall in one of my examining rooms upon which are hung the memorabilia of the 33 years since I got my medical degree. My medical diploma is there, of course. Its glass is marred by a great crack as a result of its being broken when I moved to Florida 25 years ago. I always thought I would get it fixed, but time passes pretty quickly, as you know. I have now, for thus the brain works, become fond of the crack. I see it as the same crack that

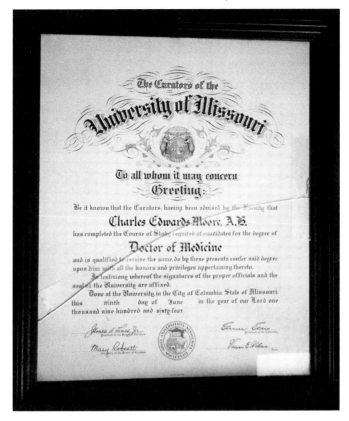

Diploma with cracked glass.

occurred in Marcel Duchamp's masterwork, "The Bride Laid Bare by the Bachelors Even," when it was found shattered after having been in storage in some shed up in Connecticut. That interesting work is now displayed in the Philadelphia Museum of Art, its message all the more potent for its cracked glass. More latterly, I have seen in the cracked glass of my diploma a metaphor for the relationship between our profession and the managed care monster. I will not, now, ever replace that piece of glass, for in my mind it has worn deeply those and other messages, reminding one that outcomes are quite uncertain.

Also on that wall are scattered pictures and letters: a perfectly beautiful young lady, in her bridal gown, whom I "reconstructed" at age 23 when, during her engagement, she required a mastectomy for cancer and subsequently something to give form to her lovely dress; a picture in full-florid crayola by a young man age 8 showing how he had looked "Before," when his ears stuck out, and then "After"; the skinning knife of an old country gent, who after I had done innumerable operations on his face, not to mention a "radical neck" for cancers, died at age 86 of a heart attack, and willed me his ancient Bowie knife; and of course a picture of my Mother that since childhood my sister and I have adored, a photograph equal in its glamorous portent to anything Katherine Hepburn contrived at about the same time, and which appeared in a 1941 edition of *Town and Country*. She is, of course, smoking a cigarette, which now seems so strange.

Well, I think, all of these and a good deal more will be coming down one of these days in the vaguely foreseeable future. To go where I wonder? Perhaps I had better start to develop a habit of thinking along such lines. Yes, I am entering the beginning of a time to think of discovery, or sending a few reconnoitering electrons down new circuits, to begin probing for those places waiting in the brain's darkness to be found and set aglow. I wonder if it is really true that those who go too suddenly from the brightly lit pathways of their professional careers into a sudden dark, unprepared, are indeed at higher risk of some nasty infarction that ironically may greet their well-earned retirement. One must strike a few lights out there in the darkness, to lead one along.

And so I shall begin.

Good grief, maybe I could take up golf! I wonder if even I, too, could hit a little ball into a hole with a stick!

THE WORLD IS NOT COMING TO AN END— NOT QUITE YET!

The other day, suiting up for surgery and putting shoe covers over my distant feet—grown farther away since my hip replacements—I bent an ear to a conversation between a pair of our most respected local surgeons. These were men of experience and judgment; they were privy to the most inside information regarding the pulse of our medical community, lately a bit arrhythmic. They were even well known as shrewd business minds.

The conversation revolved around whether, at the penultimate moment, one of our larger HMOs (God bless 'em!) would survive with any panel of physicians ("Health Care Providers") whatsoever because negotiations had broken off between our local physicians' association and this HMO. These negotiations had been much reminiscent of those good old days when hard ball was played by Unions vs. Managers, and everyone accused each other of faithlessness in the process.

Would a strike occur? Would Government step in? Thrilled as always, newspapers wrote feverish editorials that people read a little bit, threw away, and promptly forgot.

"Well, I don't know whether to sign or not," said Arthur.

"Nor I," said Al, with a happy-go-lucky grimness of countenance, and what I thought to be the merest trace of a flamboyant, but vaguely dismissive gesture.

"We don't even have a schedule for reimbursement," said Arthur.

"No one knows," said Al, "and until I know I'll never sign." He paused, "or maybe I'll sign just a little bit." This sounded odd from Al, who is known

343

for understanding real Reality from false Reality, and doing nothing by little bits.

"Good idea!" said Arthur, "I think I'll sign 'just a little bit,' too."

Having put my shoe covers on, and always liking very much to follow
leaders I respect, I piped up "I'm going to sign just a tiny bit myself, but I
think with disappearing ink."

In the operating room, while closing a nasty bedsore on a paraplegic I
have been closing them on for years and years, I pondered all that I had
overheard.

I drew a line with my marking pen, as we plastic surgeons must, and
thought to myself of the fate of private medical practice and that about this
issue, as so many others, "we see as through a glass darkly." I was given the
Xylocaine with epinephrine, which I injected here and there, at the same time
rejecting the "glass darkly" bit as having been rendered sadly trite by overuse.

One of the nicest things about surgery, which other physicians don't get
such a chance to savor, is that it is calming, even restful. You are doing something that requires a pleasant bit of concentration, bringing you sometimes
to a state of almost Zen-like involvement with the Universe, time flying by,
without the onerous responsibilities of cajoling patients, dictating charts,
signing contracts, or reading a mess of mail from lawyers. Beyond those
facts, I always feel fortunate that I get to do almost all of my surgeries all by
myself, so I do not have to present some image, bravado or jocund as the
case may be, to some other surgeon. That, of course, is simply my perception, my habit; and I beg you not to think I am stating some universal "truth"
any more valid than what you might read on any printed page, especially
your own newspaper or at least ours.

I took out the ulcer, which as usual bled like crazy because of all the scar
tissue. I took the biggest, shiniest osteotome (or is it a chisel?) and ham-
mered out the ischial tuberosity. This is a kind of orthopaedic act that quite
thrills me. It is the only time in my life that I ever get to use a little bone

wax, and as I press it onto the bleeding bone with my thumb I have the happy sensation I am doing something really good in the Universe; stanching its blood loss, and at the same time and as I press and mold it, I have a vaguely creative feeling, as though I am almost sculpting something.

Now, for the flap.

As I lift it, there is time once again for Philosophy. If Al and Arthur do not know what is happening to us, who does? Our realities are shifting beneath our feet like sand, an image as overused as "through a glass darkly." We are all of us becoming lawyers, twisting whatever we can find of truth and reality into our own image, and hoping it will win our case.

We once could take comfort in the Great Truth that ours is a "healing profession," honorable and proud; we may so indulge ourselves still, but even that is now used against us, and is merely our own wistful perception, for the bureaucrats and HMOs see us only as ciphers in an economic and public relations spreadsheet.

Oh, lovely flap! My patient will never walk again, but there is comfort in the hope that he will not have a big hole in his bottom, that something may be achieved! I rotate it around, and throw in a big mess of stitches. It is so pleasant to get the skin beautifully together so that the staples are mere "decoration," a reward to the surgery as the case comes to a close.

I call out for the Eschmann blade, with which I vastly prefer taking a skin graft over all other instruments. The compressed air-driven Reese makes a great rackety sound, and requires some running about to get it functioning. The Eschmann is a simple, quiet instrument that you can put in your pocket and take with you anywhere in case a skin graft might be needed. Perhaps it is just my perception, not any sort of "truth" at all, but it seems to me it is much easier to carry around an Eschmann dermatome than it is a five-foot-tall tank of compressed CO_2. I take my graft, gratified that it comes up so nicely, causing the nurses to give me a brief glance of admiration, batting ever so slightly their long eyelashes.

I feel relaxed. The telephone has not rung once in here. The temperature and humidity are perfect. The company is superb. There is Mozart wafting about the room. I am not being rained upon. I have enjoyed the company of the nurse anesthetist, Cynthia, whom I admire, and who shares with me our deep faith and closet understanding that if one must be somewhere in the Universe, we might as well be here. The anesthesiologist is out having coffee; but, of course, he is a good guy, too.

I run the graft through the mesher, something I do myself because it is a treat. I think how glad I am to be doing what I am doing. The contracts will sort themselves out. The HMO will survive even though it has come close to terrible deadlines. The Tallahassee Physicians Association will very likely become a defunct entity, having failed in its contractual bids. But another entity, or acronym, will after all arise, and succeed in getting the bid despite minimal differences between its bargaining position and what had been our own. If not, I am told (on good authority!) that the Governor himself might intervene, to inform all parties concerned that "something" positive had better happen so that his state employees would have health care—or else. Who knows what the realities are?

I staple the graft in place—another bit of fun—and put scarlet red on it. I like scarlet red because no one uses it, it is a beautiful color, works like magic, is cheap enough to escape banishment from the HMO's list of excluded formularies, and reminds me of Scarlett O'Hara. I picture her having invented it, and that in the true sequel to the book she made a fortune in it and other pharmaceuticals found in the rich, red earth of Georgia, and so won Rhett back to live happily ever after.

Such are my realities, truths, and perceptions. Beyond these, I risk believing it to be true that doctors will remain, surely, as some necessary ingredient in the erstwhile hopes and needs of suffering humanity, even as interpreted by government agencies and HMOs. Yes, I will sign the contract, even with real ink. But maybe I will follow up with a letter telling them I have to take it back if they do not behave.

Tonight my daughter and I are going to go out and look at the lunar eclipse. It will be delicious to watch something that so neatly blends perception and reality; and to know, as well, that the world is not coming to an end, not quite yet!

DEATH OF A COUNTESS

As a youngish person, I once read of a grand, French countess, well known for her beauty, elegant in an elegant age, and surrounded by every comfort and convenience. I regret that beyond those facts I know nothing of her except that she committed suicide, and in the note she left, explained the shocking act as being the result of an overwhelming exhaustion with life's trivial details. She has, despite the vast separation between us in time and place, affected my life, and done me good for which I thank her.

The devil, as is rightly said, lies in the "details." The details confront us every day, and without putting too fine a point upon it, I am willing to apply to those details the adjective "homely."

Regard! Even the most rich and powerful, even the most beautiful and seductive among us, must live, for example, with the repetitive details of our body's functioning. It is nastily said, and tiresomely too, come to think of it, that even the Queen of England must now and again take a four letter word. The Good, the Bad, & the Homely all itch occasionally, indeed not infrequently, and, some may argue, almost constantly. It is indeed quite enough to drive you mad, no matter how lovely the chateau in which you live, how gorgeous the portraits of your ancestors on the wall, how beautiful the Louis 15th furniture with which you are surrounded; not to mention the pleasant park and gardens without, nor the long drive from the gatehouse, winding through pleasant woods where deer gaze inquisitively at your carriage. Alas!, as the philosophers tell us, behind the facade lies the reality with which we must live and die.

But do not misunderstand my gist: I am not denying that "reality" does not bless us here and there with grand moments of exaltation, beauty, joy, and so forth. These happen now and then, but they come often unexpectedly and last but briefly. One of the reasons orgasms are so popular in our culture, even to the point of being publicly extolled on the covers of slick magazines and glorified by talk show hosts, is that for a brief second they give us the illusion that we are lifted apart from the humdrum, exalted indeed, capable of bursting at our seams, capable even of creation, inadvertent though it may be. We cannot, however, go around having orgasms all the time. And even they, to judge from what I read on those slick magazine covers promising articles within demonstrating how to have one, maybe are more occasional than one might think. It is a point I am pleased to leave alone.

The fact is that in their details our lives spin out in pretty homely fashion. And so also do our careers unless, perhaps, you are a great movie star. These people, I think more than any other group, are chosen by The Great Attractor for the great blessing of being exalted, as was the Countess herself, to what amounts to our latter day aristocracy. But despite the money, the fame, the glamour, and a good deal of leisure too, I think even Julia Roberts herself may itch now and again. The details of life are inescapable, and only briefly capable of subversion in the excitement of that orgasm or the fitting out of your private Boeing 707 (or whatever) with playpens for your child.

But at least in this career, idol that you have become, you get to escape from your itches not only as a result of all your money, but as well through the lavish trappings of romance that are built about you. How often have I thought that if only I had a mighty orchestra following me about, and a team of editors to clip away the bad parts, and a veritable Director, I might myself, just possibly, be itchless. And how marvelous in the spring, fulfilling your greatest fantasy, to surround yourself with the rich panoply of your role as Elizabeth I, *hautbois*, et al. And then, in the fall, to be a grumpy old man opposite Sophia Loren!

My own fantasy role would be to play the hero's part, a little like Ronald Reagan, as a young, handsome, charming, courageous naval officer, dive bombing down upon the Japanese fleet at Midway; and yet comforted by the secure knowledge that it was only acting, that I would survive unscathed, and at the end be given a check for a few million dollars.

Secondary to orgasms, in practical terms, film gives more people the most exultation at the most affordable price.

We crave romance; and even those who merely seek money do so at least in part for the romance that surrounds it. We cannot all be Mel Gibson or Julia Roberts, and have an entire industry bathing us in streams of glory. Indeed, if in our careers can be found some relatively smallish figment of romance and meaning, one can feel quite blessed. For those people who cannot, and who must toil daily at their repetitive tasks, which may be neither gratifying nor in the least "romantic," we must acknowledge a considerable admiration that more do not follow in the footsteps of the Countess herself.

I wish accordingly to honor herein, in some way perhaps in these essays as a whole, the ability of all of us all to withstand the homeliness of our lives. Although the devil may be in the details, and the damnable, petty ongoingness of them, we can also find in them, if you will but nudge your way further just a little, angels too. Invariably, however, you must work your way through a few devils first before you begin to discern Winged Beings who, as the poet Richard Wilbur so wonderfully put it, "swoon down into so rapt a quiet that nobody seems to be there."

I have no experience of why medical students may drop out of the curriculum. Perhaps there is no common pattern, but I permit myself the belief that many do so because "it is not what they thought it would be." Nothing, I think, is ever what you might think it might be. Our reality, after all, is supposed to be made up of quarks, which are certainly not what we think they are. We must come to terms, and in right homely fashion too, with doubt.

I know this from my experience as a surgeon, and even from my brief one as a naval aviator. For yes, as a result of my keen fantasy respecting the winning of World War II in the Pacific by single handedly dropping a bomb on the largest of the Japanese aircraft carriers, going on from there to win the heart of the heroine after steaming victoriously back into San Francisco Bay to the stirring strains of an appropriate orchestra, I applied for flight training after graduation from college. I was accepted, and, after a brief stint in blimps, duly reported to the Naval Air Station in Pensacola, Florida. By the fourth month, I had pursued enough of the course to just barely begin to think that flight training "was different from what I thought." Coincidental to this uncomfortable revelation, I was hauled up before some ophthalmologist, who rechecked my eyes and found them a fraction off caliber.

I was peculiarly undisappointed. Almost with a sense of shock, I found myself ever so faintly glad to have thus honorably escaped the rigid formalities of sitting in a cockpit, with a headache, the sun in my eyes, the yammering of the engine in my ears, and my stomach slightly queasy with the smell of oil after doing a loop. And so I served in the "fleet" a couple of years, and upon discharge had to decide what to do with my life.

"Oh God!, what can I do that will lift me out of myself, and provide romance ongoing forever?"

I decided to be a doctor, indeed a surgeon, for in surgery lay a certain rich and romantic history. I took the premed courses, meanwhile absorbing the histories of the great surgeons, their incredible deeds of derring do, the risks, the romance indeed, the intrigue, and the mystery of the human body as it was illuminated by the skillful steel of the scalpel! Throughout medical school the fire flickered some, but I fanned it, and fed it, and afterwards was off to Newfoundland and the harsh loveliness of its south coast, and from thence to East Africa in the very footsteps of Livingston.

But beyond these places, the romance of plastic surgery had called: I was deeply affected by the books of Dr. Ralph Millard, displaying the brilliant work of Sir Harold Gillies in the First World War, when overwhelming numbers of young men presented with their faces blown away. Four years of general surgery, and two of "plastic" later, and I was ready for . . . well, one settles down, falls in love (romance enough!), has a family, borrows money, pays mortgages, and develops a portfolio of insurance policies with ever-increasing premiums.

And so, after 25 years of not particularly repairing the shattered faces of youth idealized, but attending instead to concerns perhaps more prosaic and repetitive, I have this to say: that in each repetition, in each individual, there is a magical difference. Nothing and no one is the same. Every detail is always different and with its own fascination. Those details become endowed with all the magic of a Dürer painting of a bit of grass or rabbit's fur, or of an Emily Dickinson poem. It is all so different from what I had ever thought or imagined. What is more, in a curious way, it is also rather better too.

As you clearly note in these essays, I am not, any more than most of us, sustained by any sort of symphony orchestra, or brilliantly written script with all the homely or awkward parts edited out. Although I would like to cast myself, after the fashion of television stereotypes of the plastic surgeon as young, handsome, filthy rich, and a bit of a dilettante, none of this whatsoever applies. The reality is utterly different from the dream that came before it.

And so are the details, which in spite of the devil within are worth the grasping, even perhaps to find a fascination regarding.

It is too bad that the countess could not contrive it.

DÉNOUEMENT

I see that "dénouement" is a perfectly good American word; I find it in Webster's Dictionary. Of course it means the "unraveling," or the point at which the final solution is achieved, the loose ends brought together, which seems to me on the other hand quite contradictory to "unraveling." Never mind. In this dénouement, I would like to mention a few things that will I hope "bring together" to some degree the otherwise random plethora that this series of casual essays describes over the eight years of writing them.

I realize that nothing described herein relates to the extreme in terms of the practice of medicine and its dramatic—evenly highly dramatic—opportunities. What the television shows do not tell you, for their ratings would plummet if they did so, is that the practice of medicine, like life itself, is as much humdrum as it is also miraculous. Within the commonplace details of every interaction with the patient, within every second in each of our lives, reside magic and marvel. One must learn to perceive that magic, to relish its miracle, and by its study and appreciation broaden ever further one's gratitude for the opportunity life gives us. This is not the kind of "high drama," richly laced with righteous indignation and sex, that can be compressed into a half hour on *ER*. It is, on the other hand, what most fairly sane people prefer most of the time. If, as it may suit one's taste, interest is arrested here and there by variations on the theme, and something a little creative is permitted to sneak in, and even now and again a touch of drama with a happy outcome, why so much the better.

But "drama" is not something the physician particularly aspires to the cultivation of any more than the airline pilot to the desperation of an in-flight emergency, a landing with the wheels up, or two engines flaming out. We trust experience to be ready to deal with such emergencies, but just as the patient would rather not have the emergency thrust upon himself or herself, so the physician would just as soon not have to rise, in these parlous, litigious times, to the occasion very frequently.

Never mind the eight years of these essays. In the 35 years that I have been a physician, although I have wrung my hands on perhaps weekly occasions, I have experienced a few episodes that stand out, and regarding which I harbor a secret pride; there are a good deal fewer, thank goodness, respecting which I nurture a secret shame. Each of us, no matter what our walk of life, bears within us our own repertoire of unforgettable images: I will never forget the tear that occurred in the aorta of the patient who was described, perhaps a little perversely, within "Good." I will never forget the high drama of taking the young lady who had a ruptured ectopic pregnancy, on that "wild and stormy night," from Furby's Cove out of Hermitage Bay and around Connaigre Head, and so to the little cottage hospital in Harbor Britain where prompt surgery saved her life. I will never forget those billowing intestines that flew out of the young girl's abdomen in East Africa. I have always been proud that I did not faint. I will never forget the terrible time in my general surgery residency, when stressed by numerous circumstances, I simply fled; disappearing for two weeks, kneeling beside my mother, who had had a stroke that had left her utterly paralyzed, to try to find comfort for us both; and the generosity of the general surgery program that took me back, allowing me to complete my residency. The depth of the depression I felt taught me, once I had recovered from it, more than any postgraduate course in psychiatry I could have ever had. I will never forget "Old Sam," his face blown off with a shotgun, or Beatrice Herring, her face burned away in the embers of an open fire. It is a small thing, but I remember the pride I took in doing a one-stage columellar recon-

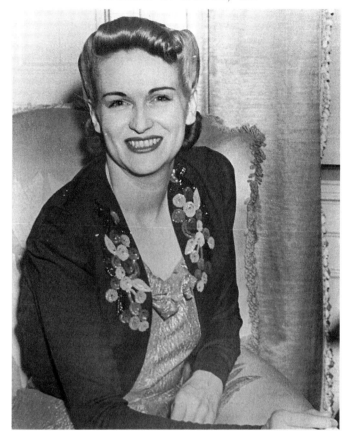

Margaret Crockett Moore (1907–1975).
My mother, whose glamour surpassed any photograph, in 1941.

struction, which I don't think had ever been described, and which I never got around to publishing a paper about. I will never forget my father's last words to me as I left his hospital room before he fell into that sweet coma which preceded his death two days later: "I'll be seeing you, kid." Beyond such fine points, I am constantly aware of the joy of these last 25 years, an office filled with its own charm, and the charm of a marvelous staff. And to come home every day, to a home I love, is beyond my words of gratitude to express.

I suppose that with perhaps only a few years left in my surgical career, I am proud that I have (almost) never been sued. The time I "more or less"

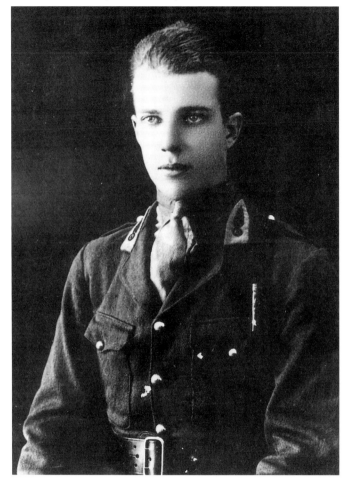

Paul Handy Moore (1898–1986).
My father, age 18, in the uniform of his regiment, the 66ième Chasseurs.

was, I did not deserve it, and the one time I maybe should have been, I was not. There is nothing of fairness or justice in the way these things happen. For what it is worth, and not to betray the meaning of a dénouement, I will mention in passing both episodes:

I should never have been sued by Ms. N., who remains, I confess it, a bit of a blot in my heart. She had been referred to me by both her psychiatrist and her dermatologist. She had intractable acne, cysts, pustules, large confluent things, which drained an odious pus. All of this, in someone who was aspiring to be an actress, or go out on a date! I saw that it would require controlling the process, before we could deal with the scars, and so, having explained to her that this would take a three-staged operative procedure to deal with, I did the first. She did well; the infections were cleared up. She never came back, and I simply heard from her lawyer, after her parents came down from the North to give me the benefits of their viewpoint, that I was being sued for having scarred her face. It never went to the courtroom, of course, and was settled for a few tens of thousands of dollars after a deposition at which I saw her a couple of years later. These things are slow. She looked remarkably better than I had ever seen her, for the scars had gone on, with time, to soften and become if not negligible much less noticeable. She was all smiles. After all the depositions, she met me out in the hall, and said that she was delighted that she had never been troubled any more by the purulent drainage. I told her, perhaps with a touch of rue in my voice, that I was glad, and we wished each other well.

But that was almost 20 years ago.

As for the boy, age 12, who died the very night I performed a repair on an accidentally cut and divided flexor tendon in his hand, I cannot apply, even now, much of philosophic comfort. He had fallen on a bottle, and the glass had cut a single tendon. Frequently this kind of thing can be postponed in its repair until the next day, more formally and sedately performed, and that is how I did it ever afterwards these past two decades. But he, coming from some distance, and his family extremely anxious to get it done, begged that it be done as quickly as possible. So we took him to the operating room. He was a slender child, what one would call. . . is the term yet still used?. . . "asthenic," pale, and a bit wan, delicate. He had been born with a congenital stenosis of the trachea, which in those days we thought people "outgrew" by the time they were four or five. I had no idea that in the anesthesiology literature, a mere six months before, an article had appeared stating how such people were at risk following general anesthesia, and that this must be guarded against. We did the surgery.

I had ordered a pain medication, which was given as a result of his complaint curiously of some pain in the abdomen, but which in retrospect probably was related to unrecognized respiratory difficulties, which led to cardiac arrest, and death. Yes, I am almost ashamed to confess that everyone else under the sun being sued, I, his veritable surgeon, was not named. This was, after all, a family I did not know whatsoever. If I had not known them before, I learned that night, literally on my knees with my arms around the shoulders of the distraught dad, and both of us weeping, how much compassion can mean! Do not think me boasting when I say that, if I have any little gift . . . and it is certainly not powerful intelligence or necessarily brilliant surgical technique . . . it is that I have been able to preserve my feelings of faith in the physician as capable of practicing compassion as well as something of science.

I suppose, as well, even in these later days of our vicissitudes, hounded by lawyers, HMOs, and our government itself, I yet can take pride in and enormously enjoy what I get to do. I realize that other specialists may find it harder. I realize that other physicians are not necessarily able to enjoy the agreeable blessing of a little office wherein work people who are far more friends than employees. Even so, it seems marvelous to me after all these years that I can yet take such pride in what I do. Medicine, and surgery, and its practice, yet remain a marvelous career, as I invariably tell young people. It is so because you know for always and ever who you are and what you do.

It may be, indeed, that I decided to become a doctor in order to gain an identity. That I should have had that insight is something I take great pride in. It has proven altogether true, and in a world where so many must seek, restlessly, shuffling papers, hoping to be this or promoted over someone else to be that, struggling to find their niche, I have been altogether spared.

When people I have never met ask me "what do you do?", I tell them "I am a physician, a surgeon in fact." This says it all, and I know nothing short of my immediate family that I am so proud to acknowledge.

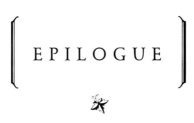

E P I L O G U E

But things are, after all, getting tough.
I would be perfectly content to stay right where I am for yet a few more
years; but, most curiously, they may not be granted. We have an HMO in
Tallahassee that I was not a part of at its inception, and will never be. For 15
years, years which found numerous newcomers moving into the specialty
field I practice within, a sort of ecological balance was struck between us
all, and the needs of our relatively small city and surrounding area. A few
years ago, the more aggressive practitioners in my field began to advertise,
a practice that has been anathema to me because we sell not a product that
can be fully known, but more a prospect, a hope, a possibility. But the affairs
of business have now been projected onto the practice of medicine, and
those forms have insidiously subverted our former "professional" ways and
means. We find ourselves now scrutinized for all manner of violations of
"proper business practice." Because, as a profession, the "benefits" of union-
ization are denied us, and out of long habit we are wary of embracing such
a practice, both for practical as well as idealistic reasons, we are accordingly
a rather easy prey for those who are practiced in the machinations of "the
business deal."

I cannot imagine that any HMO would be unaware that the physician,
who has taken an oath through thick and thin to be available to his or her
patients, to aid them in need, could turn their backs upon that oath. But
despite what you might think about doctors, and all the money they once
upon a time may have made, and the Mercedes joke that used to go around,

I believe a large number of us started out our careers as idealists; and though time and circumstance might tarnish that silver, the luster yet resides beneath the surface.

And so we carry on, as we watch our former "privileges, prerogatives," and economic well-being by the year eroded. Yes, we will keep working. But on the other hand, we may not be able to work here, or rather I may not.

For the HMO of power in Tallahassee, with which we lived in symbiotic balance has, through its own excellence and shrewd operations, suddenly gained a vast majority of our population. Patients whom I have taken care of for a quarter of a century, good friends, dear people, who join that HMO are now not allowed to see me. They, themselves, are astonished; they profess and express outrage! But the fact is that their company is now with this HMO, or they have been offered a financial savings that they simply cannot refuse for the sake of old times, be they ever so happy when weighed against their own economic need. And so, particularly in this past year and a half, I have found myself, lacking the will to advertise, and with my base of patients being thus removed from me, and expenses rising, suddenly at a loss.

I wonder at night, often enough, what to do?

Maybe go back to East Africa, I sometimes think . . .

Aside from which, might it not be fun, in a new millennium, to end at the beginning?

The Good, The Bad, & The Homely *was written by*
Charles E. Moore, MD, and edited by Carol Field. The jacket
and interior pages were designed by Mary Jane Callister / Louise Fili
Ltd, New York. Production and composition by Allison Spearman
and Jennifer Whitlow, Silverchair Science + Communications,
Charlottesville, Virginia. Printed by R. R. Donnelley in Crawfordsville,
Indiana, on 70 lb. Sterling Web Matte and set in Perpetua
and Stempel Schneidler. Published by Ardor Scribendi, New York.